Sproutin

COLOR Beginers Guide to Growing Sprouts!

Everything You Need to Know to Start Growing and Enjoying Sprouts!
Color Edition

Self-Health for Self-Help People!

Better Health for Pennies!
Superfoods You Grow Yourself!
LESS than 5 Minutes Work Per Batch!
Wonderful Nutrition for a Few Cents!
Fast Harvests: Just 4 Days from Seed to Table!
Year-Around Dirtless Farming on Your Kitchen Counter!

REVISED Color EDITION!

This is not the last word on the subject of sprouting! It's designed to be the first words to help you get started & keep you going!

By
Jim Beerstecher (Jim B!)

Copyright Page

REVISED Color CreateSpace Edition, Revised, 2017

For More Information!

For more information about this book, other books by Jim Beerstecher, arranging a personal appearance by Jim B, and the artwork of Jim Beerstecher, please feel free to contact the author via our website, www.BeginnersGuideToSprouting.com, or www.KeepItSimplePublications.com.

For additional information about sprouting, check out our web site at www.BeginnersGuideToSprouting.com

Disclaimer

This book is not intended to provide medical evaluations or advice in any sense. In this book, the author expresses his experience at reversing his own massively ill health and restoring vital living via profound changes in diet and exercise. Be sure to coordinate any changes in diet and exercise with your healthcare provider/s.

Table of Contents

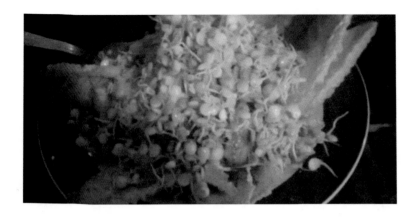

Introduction

PLEASE NOTE: Many people have suggested full color pictures would make this book a better tool for them. This, then, is that edition. I regret that the price my publishers charge for color is ridiculously high. That is with apology. The book, however is otherwise the same as the black & white edition.

Jillions of people are starting to grow their own sprouts to augment their diet, improve their general nutrition level, and enjoy better, healthier food! It's simple, easy, and *dirtlessly* cheap! Carol Finney of Richardson, Texas, quotes my perspective on sprouting, enthusiastically saying, "It's more convenient than having a tater patch in your backyard!"

In the past few years, it has become an ongoing, everyday

process that I don't even have to think about. At any given time, I have a selection of sprouts around the house in some stage of sprouting. I've gotten a good, easy routine going and share it with you in this humble book! Sprouting is a fundamental part of my health and nutrition, today!

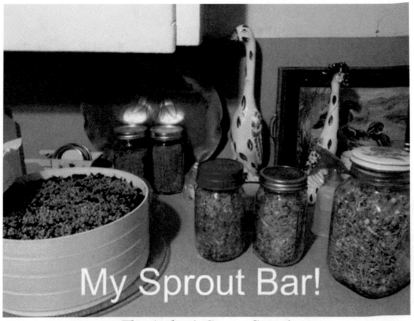

The Author's Sprout Setup!

Current conventional wisdom says that we should be eating at least 60% raw veggies and fruits in our diet, *each day!* For years I wasn't able to make that happen. The American Industrial Food Complex took over my diet early on. There was nothing vital about the food I was eating. Everything I ate was processed, chemicalized, nutritionally deficient, devitalized, and downright poisonous. That same *everything* I ate came with a lengthy and complex list of ingredients and an assurance from that same American Industrial Food Complex that all those ingredients were safe and nutritious.

In small amounts, no discernible problems were noted. Over years of consuming those things, my body began to fall apart! But, the Complex (the great American processed food production industry and their governmental counterpart, the Food and Drug Administration) denied being a part of that. They had me convinced that my problems lay elsewhere.

As I began to age, all the while eating like an American, my overall health and vitality began to devolve. My weight increased gradually for years! It was my distinct misfortune to have been obese for over 30 years! As I hit my fifties, I began to experience many of the problems of aging that my doctors assured me was just part of the aging process.

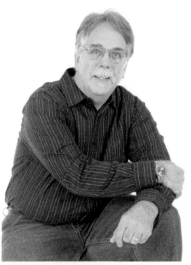

Before Sprouts! About 308 pounds!

The final straw fell after I found myself boiling over for days with a 103-degree temperature, my intestinal tract had shut down, and I was lying immobilized in a hospital bed and diagnosed with perforated diverticulitis! There I was at 300 pounds, nearly dead with a hole burst open in my intestines! My doctor assured me that 2 surgeries were all that was needed to make me as good as new! He said I didn't need to change anything about my lifestyle, that I could continue to eat and exercise (or lack thereof!) as always. I'd get a first surgery to implant a colostomy bag which would funnel all my poop out of the affected area of my colon and into a plastic bag at my side! I'd wear that thing for about a month (Now there's a fashion statement!). Then he would go in and cut out the affected foot or two of my colon, restoring my health.

I had no health insurance and very little disposable income! I was facing odds that said I'd be going bankrupt in short order... if I lived to go broke! People die of this disorder all the time. Over 30 million people have diverticulosis, little blown-out spots in their colons, which flare up from time to time and which, if burst open, can kill them quickly and with little other option. My doctor assured me that we'd caught the problem in time and I'd be on the road to health in no time (and, as he failed to mention, if I didn't die, first!)!

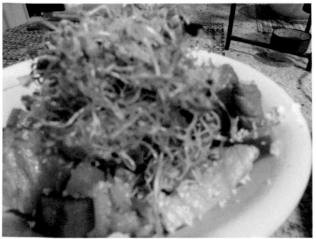

Beauty, Taste, Nutrition!
Sprouts have it all! A Baked Potato Adorned!

Along with that life-threatening problem, I was also diagnosed with Type II Diabetes, Stage 2 Hypertension, Morbid Obesity, Peripheral Neuropathy, and Major Depression! I was walking with a cane due to a bum knee, suffered from constant back pain, and couldn't pursue anything physical for more than a few minutes each day lest I spend several days in bed recovering! The list of complaints went on and on and on and on and on!

I didn't want to believe surgery was my only option. Despite his assurance that there was no other way to deal with this, I decided to look at the world of natural health and healing. As I began to review the literature available on natural foods and healing (both on the internet and in the printed media), as I began to watch and learn from all the new documentaries available on natural foods and natural healing (sites like Food Matters TV, Netflix, Amazon Prime, and the Internet in general!), I began to see a pattern. People who opted out of the American Industrial Food Complex were beginning to cure all sorts of the so-called diseases of aging! They were dancing with joy and free from long lists of so-called chronic illnesses (a chronic illness, by definition, is something you never get rid of. Boy were they wrong!)

They were overcoming all of the diagnoses I had and many others! Many illnesses thought to be directly linked to aging turned out to be directly linked to long-term exposure to the poisons and devitalized nutrients in our food chain!

Could it really be that simple?

Yes it really was that simple!!!

-

To make an already lengthy story a bit lengthier, I completely changed my diet and lifestyle. Today I no longer have any of the diagnoses listed above! As of today, in less than 2 years of eating healthy life-giving vital foods prepared in ways to optimize the nutritional values to nurture my body, here's what has been essentially cured:

- ✓ Perforated Diverticulitis, GONE!
- ✓ Type II Diabetes, GONE (A1C in normal range for over a year and a half!) with no re-occurrence of symptoms!
- ✓ Stage 2 Hypertension, GONE with normal blood pressure achieved without medication!
- ✓ Morbid Obesity, GONE! In fact, after over 30 years in some stage of obesity, *I'm no longer obese at all!*
- ✓ Peripheral Neuropathy, GONE!
- ✓ Major Depression, GONE!

And here are some other improvements I love to dance, sing, and crow about!

- ✓ I've lost over 100 pounds, so far!
- ✓ I can be physically active all day and feel great tonight and tomorrow!
- ✓ No more cane to walk with... and no need for one!
- ✓ No more back pain!
- ✓ No more medications!
- ✓ No doctors, aside from regular checkups!
- ✓ No surgeries!
- ✓ Absolutely NO more mythical diseases of aging!
- ✓ And I didn't have to go broke!

All of that was accomplished by:

1. By halting the intake of poisonous, devitalized foods!
2. By simultaneously beginning and continuing the intake of unadulterated foods: sprouts, fresh veggie juices, and eating unprocessed foods (Mostly raw!)!
3. By getting educated about all of the above from others who are similarly healing themselves!
4. Undertaking some physical exercise as I became able!

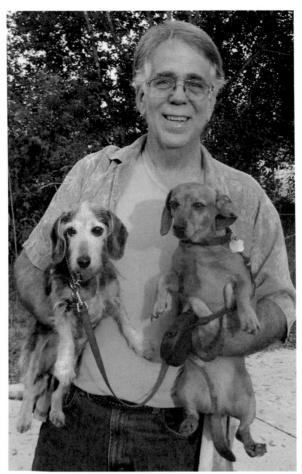

Jim lost 100+ pounds,
but still loves his weenies!

Did I go broke? Nope! These changes ended up saving me tons of money by not having to go to doctors or hospitals and by no longer buying medications, both over the counter and prescription! I also save by not buying anti-suffering aids like over the counter potions, canes, wheelchairs, and the like.

***Also, the new way of eating I discovered for
myself actually costs me far less in one day
than one trip to a fast food joint!***

Also, the new way of eating I discovered and developed for myself actually costs me far less in one day than one trip to a fast food joint! I actually eat far less food than before and enjoy every bite and slurp of real nutrition much more!

Where I had no time to prepare food, *before*, and relied on fast foods and quick-devitalized foods from the grocer, I now have plenty of extra time to prepare whole, vital food.

The five biggest changes I made were!

1. I began to grow sprouts on an ongoing basis, at home, and eat them with *every* meal!
2. I began to juice whole veggies daily!
3. I transitioned to eating only whole, unadulterated foods!
4. I learned about colon health and began to practice what I learned.
5. After a couple of months or self-repair, I worked up to aerobic exercising 3 times a week for at least 20 minutes... a task which took several months to build up to!

This book is a major part of the solution I've found to restore my health, vitality, and zest for life! It is my profound hope that you can find your own set of solutions for yourself. The help is there if you want it.

14

On to Sprouting!

I promise that if you begin to grow sprouts, that will begin to provide just that much more real nutrition to the 100+ billion cells in your body and begin a turnaround for your overall health!

Each and Every Positive Change, No Matter How Small, Adds Up!

Each little positive change you make adds up and helps you gain the strength and willingness to move on to healthier lifestyle choices.

And, for those of you who are enjoying good health already, I promise, adding sprouts to your life will aid in keeping you that way and help improve upon your already good health! *It only takes about five minutes over 4 days to grow some of the most nutritious food on the planet!*

I apologize for my zealous preaching and clamoring about my personal health revolution. I can only hope you experience such a turnaround for yourself, if need be, and that you get a chance to feel as wonderful as I now feel! Start growing and eating your own sprouts today!

Start growing and eating your own sprouts today! It only takes about five minutes over 4 days to grow some of the most nutritious food on the planet!

Put fresh sprouts on everything you eat!!!! (Well, maybe except for your organic frozen fruit sorbet, not in your hot herbal tea, and for sure not in your glass of soymilk!) Be sure to include them on your morning oatmeal, on your eggs, in fresh veggie juices, in sandwiches, on salads, in soups, in veggie loaves, over any entree, and, of course, as a delightful snack food all by themselves!

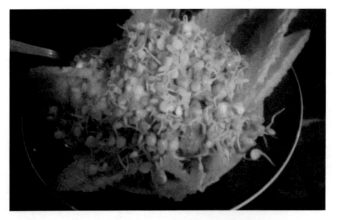

Healthy food can be sexy, too!

When a new batch of sprouts becomes ready, toss the rest of the previous batch into your juicer, including them in your daily whole foods juicing! Better still, *plan* to include fresh sprouts in every juice you make! By *plan*, I mean that you might consider sprouting a few more sprouts each week to have that extra you want for juicing.

As you move along into sprouting, please email me or write to me and let me know how this is working for you. When you have questions, ask! Be sure to include any new ideas and tips for sprouting you come across so I can add them to this little book to help others (And to allow me to thank you, personally and/or publicly!). I'll put them in the next edition and say nice things about you when I give you the credit! You can reach me at Jim@BeginnersGuideToSprouting.com.

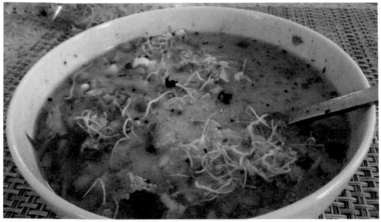

Sprouts Are Cooked in This Stew and Added When Served!

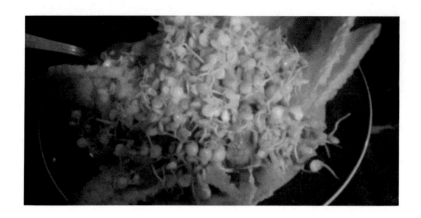

1: Healing, Healthful Living with Sprouts!

Don't Panic! The whole process of growing a 1/2-gallon batch of nutritious health-restoring sprouts takes only about 5 minutes!

And that five minutes is spread out over about a week!

Simple, easy, cheap, and outrageously nutritious!

I don't even think about growing sprouts any more. It's just part of the kitchen routine. I always have at least one jar or tray of sprouts in process. I usually have a gallon plastic food storage bag lying about on the kitchen counter greening up a bit. In everything I prepare to eat, whether cooked or raw, I'm always grabbing some sprouts to toss into or on top of.

I think sprouts must be about the most nutritious food source available. A dormant seed springs to life and converts all the stored energy into life-giving and plant building biochemicals, nutrients to sustain a new life. When I eat a handful of these nutritional powerhouses, every cell of the over 100 million cells in my body get all excited. I feel a bit of a rush when I am eating sprouts. Try it and you'll understand soon enough, too!

Seeds, whether nuts, grains, legumes or whatever other form you find, store energy and the spark of life to create a new plant. When you eat beans, grains, nuts, or other seeds cooked or raw, you only get a tiny bit of the biochemicals essential for life. Mostly you get the energy stored as carbohydrates.

You need carbs to live, too. But in a world full of devitalized food brimming with dangerous chemistry, we have plenty of empty carbs to go around. We are sorely lacking in real nutrients, the kind of biochemicals our bodies have been utilizing for millennia but can no longer seem to get enough of.

Since the industrial revolution, we've been chipping away at the fresh, complete nutrition available in nature, leaving millions of us to live devitalized lives and die unnecessarily earlier from illnesses created from the long-term effects of such poor food.

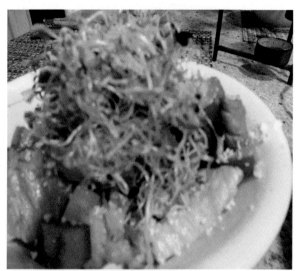

Baked Potato with Salad on Top & Sprouts for a Crown!

One simple, cheap, affordable way to begin to renew and refill your nutritional bank, your personal health, and the quality of your life is to begin to incorporate sprouts and sprouting into your daily routines.

Sprouting seeds are about as cheap a food as you can buy! One pound of organic lentils, for example, cost less than $2! That should give you about 3 gallons of sprouts! That's enough life-building and life-enriching superfood sprouts to last you several weeks! What a deal!

You're saying that you don't have the time to prepare whole foods? You say your life is too busy? You need instant pre-

prepared foods and you don't mind if the content lacks complete nutrition as long as it tastes great and provides comfort? You feel fine, you say!

In less time that it takes to drive over to a fast food joint, park and stand in line and wait or wait in the drive up window line, order some of their devitalized, chemical-laden food, check out and pay, and drive home... you can have the most healthy food on the planet! Yep, in less than 5 minutes a week, you can grow all of the sprouts you can eat! That five minutes is spread out over the week, so you have to wait a few days for the first ones to grow. After that, this book will show you how to maintain that ongoing stream of the healthiest food on the planet! All for only about five minutes a week! Imagine having an ongoing stream of whole, vital, living food ready to eat at a moment's notice!

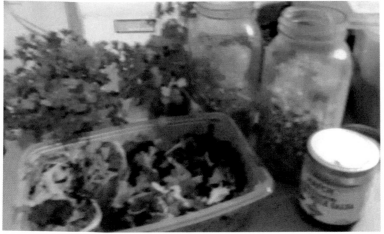

My Salad Bar with Loads of Sprouts1

Five minutes to get started! And using my system, you don't have to go out of your way or drive anywhere. You do it right on your kitchen counter next to your sink. So, twice a day, when you are putting a bowl in the sink or getting a glass of water, you can take 15 seconds to rinse your sprout batch. And since it's on the counter right in front of you, you don't have to worry about forgetting them. They'll remind you!

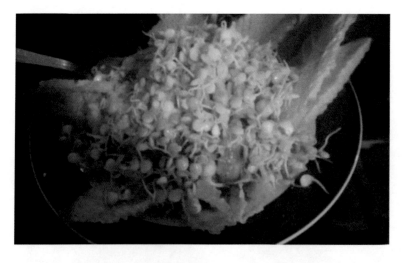

Romaine Lettuce Topped with Lentil Sprouts!

Getting started will take a bit more effort. You'll have to go get a sprouting jar, sprouting trays, or make your own sprouting jar with jars and cheesecloth. Then you have to go get something to sprout. I suggest you just get a pound of lentils to get started. They are everywhere and you don't have to go out of your way to get them. If it doesn't work out for you, you haven't lost much and you can make lentil soup out of the remaining lentils you didn't try to sprout.

Just start. Just try to get one batch going. That's all I ask of you. Once it gets done, you can decide if you can handle the effort again. Even if you forget to start more sprouts, you can always start more when you remember. Just keep trying.

And once you see that batch come to life, once you pop a bunch in your mouth and begin to chew, once your body begins to clamor for more sprouts, you, too, will be hooked on the healthiest food I know of!

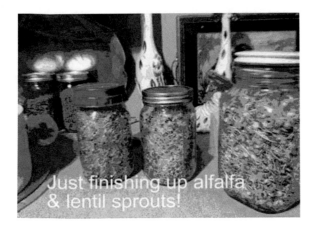

Sprouts: The Best Food I Know!

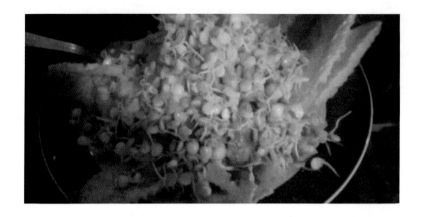

2: What Sprouting Is!

Quite simply, sprouting is causing seeds, nuts, grains, and beans to begin to grow. When a seed germinates and sprouts, it takes a dormant pod and creates all the nutrients vital to create a living plant! So, a newly sprouted seed, bean, grain, or nut is perhaps the most nutritious food available. Sprouts can be eaten when the sprouted part is only 1/8" long! I usually try to wait until they are about one to two inches long, plus or minus.

Since sprouts are so small, sprouting means you have to sprout large numbers of small seeds. In a ½ gallon sprouting jar, for example, I use about 1/3 cup of lentils (That's a whole lot of lentils!). In about 4 to 5 days, and after a non-grueling few minutes of work on my part, I get a half gallon of wonderfully nutritious freshly-sprouted little plants to nurture the hundreds of millions of cells in my body with real, great nutrition!

I can buy a small 1-pint container of commercially sprouted sprouts at the store for about four bucks! It would take about 4 of those little plastic containers to fill up my ½ gallon jar. So, my minutes of labor yields about $16 worth of sprouts! And I know, by growing them myself, they are fresh!

It's interesting to note how valuable the process of sprouting is in an economic sense. $16.00 per 5 minutes of work translates into an hourly wage value of $192.00! Those are pretty great wages for your efforts!

But, I'm not actually working at sprouting. If I did, I could make up 12 half-gallons in about an hour of work (It would actually take less time than that!). So, for as little as it takes to get the job done, it certainly pays to sprout, both financially and nutritionally!

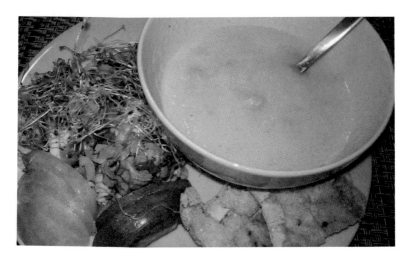

Veggie Platter! Great Eating!

What does it cost to sprout? To grow a ½ gallon of lentil sprouts costs between 15 to 23 cents, depending on the market price of your lentils!

No matter how you look at it, whether from the perspective of health, nutrition, money-savings, personal fulfillment, self confidence, or taking control of your food supply process, sprouting is a winning process to get involved in!

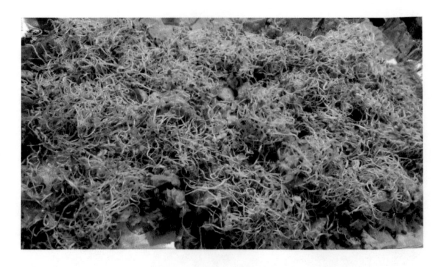

Tasty and Healthy! Nachos Covered in Sprouts!

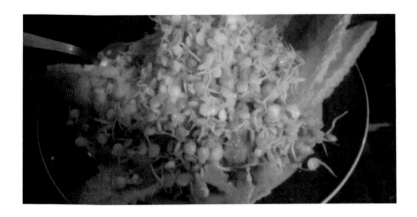

3: What Sprouting Isn't!

Sprouting is not some esoteric vegan ritual, although many vegans enjoy the process and the results! People from all walks of life enjoy sprouts. Even died-in-the-wool meat eaters enjoy sprouts with their meals!

Sprouting is not dangerous! If you follow the simple steps outlined in this book, you'll be able to produce all the fresh, wholesome, healthy sprouts you want! Like with any raw vegetable, you must watch for obvious signs of problems. But problems are rare if you follow these instructions.

Sprouting isn't a panacea! It's the first step to a healthy way of living and eating that can help you heal and grow in healthy ways, restoring your body's vitality. Just adding sprouts, alone, to your diet at every meal is bound to improve your overall health in direct proportions. It's not the only change I had to make to reverse all of my own supposedly-chronic conditions, lose 100 pounds, and restore my vitality, vigor, and health! But it is a wonderful move in the right direction!

Sprouting isn't dirty, messy, or smelly! In fact, some sprouts, like dill, have a nice savory aroma. Fresh sprouts are a bouquet of mild natural aromas.

And there's no dirt in the kitchen, either! If you decide to grow sunflower sprouts or wheat berries in dirt, you might want to put them on the back porch. But you can enjoy sprouts every day for the rest of your life and never have to mess with dirt!

Sprouting is not hard or tricky! If I can do it... you can, too. The sprouts do all the work. You just rinse a little water over them a few times each day.

Sprouting is not a new fad. People who are concerned about optimal health and optimal nutrition have been sprouting for a long long long long time! Millions of people are sprouting today! Cruising sailors, health-conscious people, and people who live away from shopping centers have been sprouting for longer than I can imagine!

I've noticed that grazing animals will always jump at a chance to grab the new shoots of freshly sprouted grasses. I always thought it had to do with the tenderness of the shoots. But today I understand that it is because their bodies, like mine, crave the concentrated nutrient levels of freshly-sprouted plants!

I'm living testimony to how well they serve us. You can be, too! Be sure to share your success and failures with us as you head on down this road. Together we can make a difference in all our lives!

Sprouting, then, isn't really anything but goodness, health, vitality, nutrition, and fun! Hard to find anything at a fast food joint that comes anywhere near close!

And, to make matters even better, sprouting IS a fast food, in that you can make a bunch up in less than five minutes of your time. So, if you are a fast food junky, you'll love sprouts!

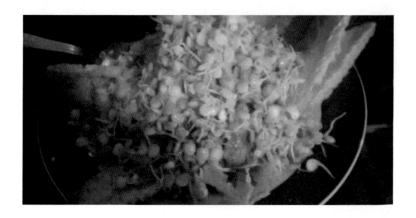

4: How Simple & Easy Sprouting Really Is!

Here are the simple steps to simply, easily, and readily grow sprouts! This chapter goes into detail on the sprouting process. At the end, I'll give you a simple outline to follow once you get going. First you get the information and understanding, then the outline.

First, Measure Out and Inspect the Dried Seeds

For a quart jar, I'll measure out and add about a quarter of a cup lentil, mung beans, or other similarly-sized, larger seeds. If I'm using alfalfa or another smaller seed, then I only add about

2 tablespoons.

For a half-gallon jar, I'll put in about a third to a half cup of dried beans or larger seeds or grains. Similarly, I'll only add about a quarter cup of alfalfa or other smaller seeds.

When you add the seeds, you'll be thinking, "That'll never get very full." In a few days, you'll be amazed. The volume expands daily. Days 4 and 5, it seems to double as the sprouts green up!

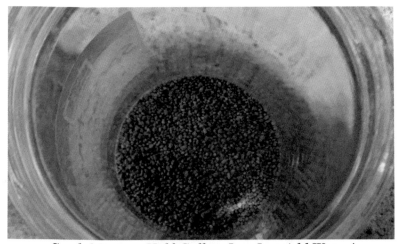

Seed Mix in a Half-Gallon Jar. Just Add Water!

It's important to sort through the seeds, prior to soaking, and pull out anything that doesn't belong there. You might find a few small clods of dirt, pebbles, sticks and twigs, or other foreign matter. Pull it out before you get started. I rarely find any foreign matter, any more. They come well sorted and gleaned. But you need to remain vigilant.

All you need to do, is be sure the seeds, beans, or grains are covered by water so they can soak up all they want overnight.

If you are living with minimum water, like aboard a cruising sailboat or out backpacking, just cover them with water. Keep an eye on them to be sure they don't soak it all up. That way you can add more water as needed.

Don't worry about wasting the water. Once you are done soaking your seeds, you can add that water to your stockpot or whatever you are cooking. You can even just drink the leftover soaking water... it's got some nutritional value and is still good drinking water.

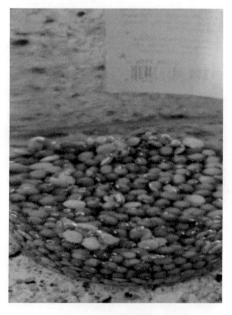

Just Add Water!

Put the Seeds in the Jar and Fill the Jar to About Half Full

(Or half empty, depending on your particular outlook!)

Fill the jar with clean filtered water, or whatever water you would use for drinking. Obviously, the best possible water should be used for personal consumption as well as soaking and rinsing sprouts.

Put the Screen Lid on the Jar and Set It Aside

Same goes for sprouting trays which will be discussed later on.

Do not set the soaking sprouts in direct sunlight. A bit of indirect sunlight doesn't seem to be a problem.

Soak the seeds for 18 - 24 hours. I usually get around to this task sometime during the day when I'm already working in the kitchen, say making breakfast or lunch. Rather than obsessing about how long they've soaked, I simply wait until sometime the next day to move ahead... no clocks, no obsessing... just wait until tomorrow! A couple of hours more or less will work just fine, too.

I've read a bunch of books and articles about sprouting over the years. They used to all say to put them in a dark place, like under the sink. Well, my "under the sink" areas aren't the nicest places to grow things you'd want to eat some day! So, I began to sprout out in the open, on my clean counter tops, but not in the path of direct sunrays.

For convenience sake, it also means I sprout on the counter top next to my sink. It's out in the open and easy to see and remind me to rinse regularly.

So let's stop with the under-the-sink model of sprouting. Trust me, there's nothing nastier than finding a dried up container of moldy sprouts under your sink a month or so after you put them there (Eeeeuuuuuuuwwwwww!!!)

So, once you put the screen lid on the jar, or cover the tray, and set it aside, the hardest work of sprouting is over. In 3 to 4 days, you'll have a nice jar full of fresh, delicious, healthy sprouts!

If You MUST Have Darkness!

OK, if you must have darkness for the developing seeds/sprouts, simply wrap or cover the jar with a fresh, clean dishtowel. That cuts the light out, but still keeps the sprouts out in the open where you can see them hiding under the dish towel and remember to deal with them those few moments a day.

I've done it both ways and don't see much, if any difference. In my RV and on my boat where there was more direct sunlight around to deal with, I usually cover loosely with a fresh dishtowel. Simple.

The Next Day

The sprouts have been soaking for 18 - 24 hours, approximately. I usually do this late morning or around lunchtime. But if you have to go to work, you can either drain them before you head out to work or when you get home. Most books, articles, and videos want to soak for 6 to 8 hours. Since this book has come out, though, it seems that a lot of others are coming on board with the overnight soaking process, thereby extending the hydration phase.

(NOTE: If you're gonna leave the sprouts to soak until you get home from work, it's often a good idea to drain the murky water and re-fill with fresh water. You don't have to. It's an option for those who prefer.)

The water your seeds are soaking in may be a bit brown from the tannins in the seed hulls (no big deal). Drain the sprout jar.

Save the water for cooking or drinking if you want. I just usually pour it on living plants. However when I was cruising on a small sailboat, I always re-used that water since fresh drinking water was at a premium. Feel free to drain the jar into a pot for cooking, as there is some nutritional value to the water.

Rinse and drain your sprouts again, once or twice, with tap water. Comfortable temperatures seem to work best for me. If it's too hot or cold for me, it's probably too hot or cold for my little seeds. The little seeds or beans are looking for spring conditions to sprout. Help them along with comfortable water temps.

Turn the Jar on its Side, and Gently Roll It Around a Couple of Times

… once the water is drained out, of course!

With smaller seeds, like alfalfa, the seeds will sort of stick to the walls of the jar ensuring they get good aeration and drainage. The bigger seeds, like mung beans, will just clank and flop around in a friendly way (again, no big deal).

Another reason to turn the jar a few times a day is to keep the sprouts from getting moldy. By moving them around, they get exposed to fresh air and excess water moves around rather than getting stagnant.

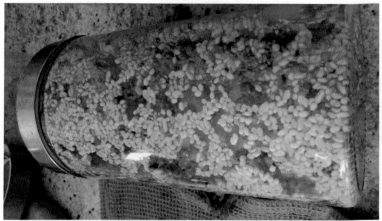

After Initial Soak, Drain, Roll, and Carefully Lay on Side

Keep Your Sprout Jar Next to Your Kitchen Sink

That way, when you are at the sink to rinse a dish, wash something, or get a glass of water, you can take about 7 seconds and give the sprouts a quick rinse.

Try to rinse your sprouts two or three times a day, when you're at the sink and you think about it. Keep the jar or tray out in the open next to the kitchen sink to remind you. Even if you're covering it with a fresh dishtowel, you'll see it hiding out there in plain site and be reminded to rinse them.

Be sure to run the water gently, too. These are delicately unfolding seeds and need gentle treatment at all times to keep from damaging their germinating efforts. Easy does it, when handling your sprouting setup.

Gently Set the Jar Down, Out of Direct Sunlight

You've just finished your second big day as a sprout farmer. Blistering work, eh?

Be sure to rinse and drain at least 2 times a day (3 or 4 times in the summer!). It doesn't take a written schedule, either. As long as they get a little drink of water a couple of times a day, they'll be happy and grow well!

Days 3, 4, and 5

Two or three times a day, fill the jar to just over the sprouts' level with fresh, clean water and let it sit in there a few seconds.

Drain, rotate the jar to spread out the seeds and young sprouts, and set it back down gently. Re-cover if you are doing it that way.

Sprouting days like this will require upwards of 30 seconds of your time! Can you handle the pace? It takes far less time to grow a batch of fresh sprouts than it does to read about growing them. Weird, eh?

Let's say you forgot to rinse the little fellas in the morning and now it's six o'clock in the evening. You've just gotten home from work and they seem to be bone dry. When you rotate the jar, you hear what sounds like grains of hard sand clacking against the jar.

What now? When that happens, I'll fill the jar to just above the sprout level and let them soak for a while (Anywhere from 5 minutes to a half hour should do it). Then, drain them, roll the jar and set them back down to continue sprouting. No worries!

By soaking a bit longer on the first day, the sprouts get a bit more water momentum. They won't die if they miss a water/rinse. But given a few extra minutes to soak a bit, they'll pop right back into the program.

Oh, FYI, you don't have to sit and watch them soak, either. That would increase the time to grow them. More importantly, the sprouts can soak just fine on their own.

After Day 2, (Let's Call It Day 3) You Can Actually Begin to Eat Most Sprouts

Gently grab a pinch of them out of the jar or tray and pop them into your mouth. You'll begin to develop your pallet for sprouts. You'll learn to enjoy the subtle differences in taste and texture that different sprouts produce. You may decide to harvest sprouts based on shorter lengths for things like baking breads and adding to soups and longer ones for salads, sandwich toppings, etc.

Generally, I just let them get bigger. I usually wait until the length of the individual sprouts is about 1" to 2" before I start eating them in full measure. That insures some chlorophyll has been made and I have the largest percentage of great usable nutrients growing in the seeds.

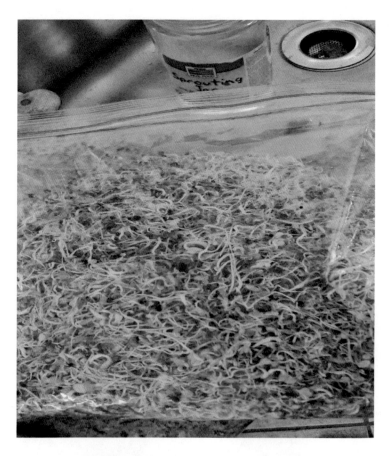

Sprouts before Greening for a Day!

Sometimes, I'll leave them to get to about two-and-a-half inches. If they get too long, so they begin to taste and feel too leggy, or tough, just toss them into the juicer! Sprouts are *all* good!

When I don't have any sprouts in the fridge, I'll often toss a bunch directly from the growing jar or tray into something I'm fixin' in the kitchen! Any sprouts are good sprouts (Well, of course, except for slimy ones... we'll talk later!)!

On the Last Day or Two

I make sure the sprouts are able to get some good indirect light or maybe an hour or two of direct yellow beams of sunlight. That helps to get the chlorophyll process going, making them healthier for you. I call it *"Greening them Up!"* (Catchy phrase, eh?)

In my kitchen, they may be six feet or more from a window and there may not be any sunrays shining directly into the kitchen. But they still green up! The little sprouts find enough light to create *greenage*!

Chlorophyll production is a wonderful process! It adds to the nutritional value of your sprouts as well as the aesthetics!

Let's Review!

You soaked one day, watered / rinsed / drained two or three times a day for two or three days more.

Now it's time to begin to eat them in earnest!

This is the best part!

With beans like lentils, mung beans, chickpeas, black-eyed peas, and the like, I just rinse them well and put them in a plastic tub or zip bag and toss them into the fridge.

You can leave the bag open a bit to keep them fresh, alive, and keep them from spoiling. If you keep them closed up in the fridge, just be sure to open them up once a day to get some fresh air.

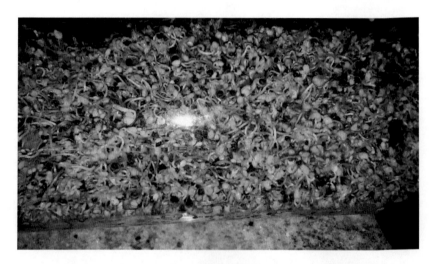

Just an Afternoon in Indirect Sunlight Greens them Up a Lot!

Remember, they are still alive! You can even pull the open bag out and set it on the counter every couple of days to let them get some light and fresh air. Rinse them and drain if they seem to be drying out.

It's fun to watch a half full-bag of sprouts re-fill itself by leaving it out on the counter, slightly open, for a day!

Pull out sprouts when you need them. Making a sandwich? Pull out a healthy pinch and place on top right before you crown the top piece of bread!

Got a soup cooking? Pull out some sprouts and toss them in! You can dice them up, too, if you prefer. When you serve the soup later, drop a pinch on top to make the presentation more gourmet looking and feel the fresh crunch when you chew!

Making a salad? Cover the top with a half inch, or more, of sprouts. OK, I've been told by newbies that a quarter-inch layer is a better way to get started with sprouts on top of a salad. It doesn't overwhelm the rest of the salad ingredients as much. But, if you're like me, in short order, you're gonna be piling them on.

You'll catch on. I even put sprouts in my veggie juices! I use a slow-speed, masticating juicer to preserve the biochemicals in my fresh juices. But whatever juicer type you use, include your sprouts, too, for added nutrients!

Don't be bashful! When I first got started sprouting, I was guilty of the same thing, myself. I would count out a very few sprouts and add them to my food sparingly, at best. Sprouts are *not* an endangered species! You are growing them for pennies and there are lots more where these came from. So pile them on! Practice using more and more in everything.

If the sprouts are in the fridge a couple or three days, it's a good idea to give them a bit of a rinse, when you think about it, just to keep them fresh. Remember to drain well! With larger batches, I'll let the bag sit on the counter for five minutes or so just to let the excess water drain to the bottom of the bag or container. That makes it easier to insure they don't drown later.

If they begin to get gooey and smelly, it's time for the compost or, if you have them, your chickens. Usually, they get eaten sooner. Never toss them in the trash... composts and chickens both love sprouts, too! My chickens used to fight over the sprout scraps!

A Bit More About Alfalfa Seeds and Other Small Seeds!

Alfalfa seeds and many other small seeds have brown cellulose seed casings that fall off and just sit there during the soaking and sprouting process. They'll get between your teeth and make people wonder about your oral hygiene. It makes my teeth look like a poppy seed bagel!

I don't know how many times I've popped a pinch of sprouts from the sprouting jar to my mouth. Right after, grinning in the mirror, I'd see hoards of little dark splotches in all the crannies of my teeth and gums! What a site!

So, when it's time to harvest your little alfalfa sprouts, sprout mixes, and smaller seeds, put the whole mess in a large pot and flood it with water. From there, pull out handfuls of sprouts, gently moving them about before lifting them out of the water to be sure you get rid of the majority of the little brown hulls. That's it. It might take a whole minute to process a half-gallon of sprouts that way... but it will save you three days of extra tooth brushing!

And this is an optional step as the casings are fine to eat (More fiber!). Just be to check your teeth often after sampling sprouts!

The rinsing process also gets rid of small unsprouted seeds, too! Even the best seed stock will have some seeds that just don't sprout.

You'll be amazed at how much better your sprouts feel and taste in your mouth with all that "other material" gone, too. They look fresher and greener and actually feel better in your mouth!

And Now... Making This an Ongoing Process

This is a biggie, y'all! I sprouted now and then for years. I'd maybe sprout a half dozen times a year. When cruising in my sailboat in more remote areas, I'd sprout regularly to help supply fresh produce.

Most of the books I read on the subject covered it nicely. But they failed to include a plan of action to make sprouting an ongoing activity. If you don't sprout, you don't get to keep eating them and enjoying them and enjoying improved health and vitality that they bring. So it's absolutely crucial for you to make this an ongoing activity to get the most out of this wonderful food!

Here's the plan: When you harvest some sprouts, immediately after removing them from the jar or tray, clean the jar or tray with dish soap and water and put the next batch of sprouts on to soak. That's it! No magic! Simple! Easy! Cheap! It works if you will just do it. To repeat: Once you harvest a batch of sprouts, immediately start a new batch. Simple.

The Big Secret: Immediately after removing a batch of sprouts from the sprouter, clean the sprouter and put the next batch of sprouts on to soak!

The process I follow is to sprout enough sprouts to keep me eating sprouts three meals a day until the next batch comes in. So, the jar should always be on your counter in some phase of sprouting something. If you live alone you might get by with a quart jar. If you live alone but eat a lot of sprouts, you might need a half-gallon jar. Or you might do well with 2 jars for more variety day-to-day. If you live in a couple situation, a half-gallon jar might fit better. Got a batch of kids, too... get several half-gallon jars going. You can expand this process and deflate it as your needs and desires change.

In 2014, I spent the first 8 months of the year traveling in a bubble-top van motorhome (AKA a Class B RV) around the eastern half of the USA. During that time, I kept my sprouts going full time. It was simple and easy and I did it exactly the way I've described in this book.

I've done the same thing for months at a time in a Catalina 22 sailboat, a boat that is so small, you can't even stand up in it! I really believe you can grow wonderful sprouts in any living situation you find yourself in.

Whether you use jars, bags, or trays... just get started sprouting today. It's not rocket science. It certainly doesn't take a lot of effort or time or money, either! The results are overwhelmingly wonderful for you, too!

That's it! Simple! Easy! Cheap! Delicious and Nutritious! Self-Health for Self-Help people!

Self-Health for Self-Help People!

(Say *that* five times really fast! I tried, can't do it!)

As promised, here's the quickie outline...

5-Minute Sprouting Process

Day 1: Put sprouts on to soak

Day 2: Drain, rinse, & drain. Then rotate the jar and lay out on the counter.

Day 3: Rinse, drain, and lay out on the counter.

Day 4: Rinse, drain, and lay out on the counter.

Day 5: Rinse hulls out, drain, bag and refrigerate. Clean your sprouter and repeat beginning right now!

Early Harvesting Notes

Before you bag your sprouts and put them in the fridge, even during the third and fourth days of sprouting, you can begin eating them right out of the sprouting jar, bag, or tray.

Beginning at the end of the second day, you can pull some out of the jar and toss them into whatever food you are preparing or just enjoy them as a tasty snack!

If you run low on supply, you can keep pulling them out of the jar as they grow. You'll discover an interesting phenomenon about sprouting. You can pull out about a third of the total yield, and, by keeping them sprouting a day or two longer than a normal batch, you'll still have a full jar of sprouts for a yield! How does it know? Truth be told, the individual sprouts will be a bit larger, but just as good in every respect! What a wonderful economy of nutrition!

DO NOT try this method of extending your supply with a fast food hamburger. It just won't work. Don't try it with a steak, either. Nor will it give you anything but grief with ice cream... even those single-serving half-gallon containers I used to suck down in an evening.

DO TRY IT with your fresh, homegrown sprouts!

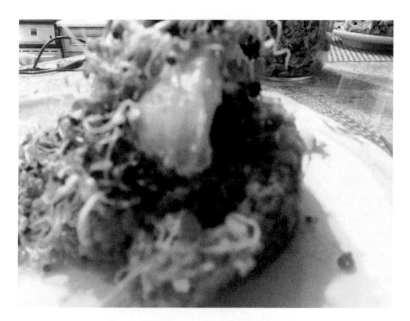

Better than Any Restaurant I Know!

Nature seems to really know what she's doing... if we'll just listen, learn, and practice! That's really the essence of sprouting, listening to nature and learning from it.

It's a good time to try something new. Like they say in the halls of all the 12-step groups out there, "Nothing changes if nothing changes." It's this little change in your diet, in your relationship with food, that will help you change your life.

What To Do With Extra Sprouts

If you slow down on consumption, no problem. Occasionally you'll end up with a surplus of sprouts. Put some in a baggy and give them to friends and family. Sprouts are a great homegrown gift!

Also, if you get too many, just juice them in your normal veggie juicing.

Remember to use the pulp left from juicing in everyday cooking. Add it to soups, breads, stews, veggie burgers & loaves, and whatever strikes your fancy.

I generally take a batch of fresh sprouts to potlucks. You never know who's gonna "discover sprouts" next. And you will find you are changing lives for the better all the while making your own life better. People will sigh in amazement at seeing so many "expensive" and "gourmet" sprouts!

Spread the Health, Y'all!

I go to lots of meetings in the course of my week. I'll frequently take small bags of sprouts with me and leave them on the "cookie table." I have my card on the bags and friends are becoming conditioned to sprouts. It's helping me by helping them.

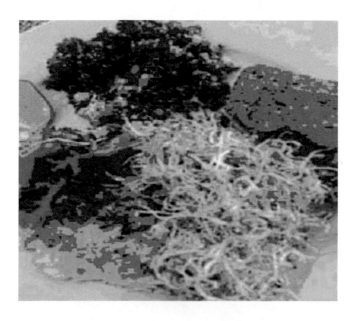

Another Wonderful Sprout Breakfast!

The above picture points out the gourmet beauty of sprouts.
Any ordinary meal, say, scrambled eggs with toast, can be made
a health fest with a gob of sprouts, a few leaves of cilantro,
some quinoa salad, and a section of lime to squeeze over it all.

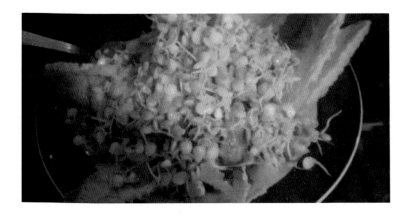

5. Sprouting Process Review

Here's a simplified review of the process with, of course, even more hints and tips tossed in!

1. Measure out seeds, beans, or nuts to sprout!

2. Spread them out and check for rocks, sticks, dirt, etc, to be sure you'll only get what you planned to get!

3. Put them in your jar or tray and cover generously with water!

4. Set them beside your sink and wait 18 - 24 hours (Overnight!)!

5. Drain the excess water and spread the spouts out in their jar or tray!

6. Place them on the counter! Cover if you prefer.

7. Two or Three times a day rinse with fresh water, drain, spread out in their container and place them back on the counter!

8. Begin eating them whenever you like after the second day! Harvest on day 3, 4, 5, or whenever they are the length you prefer!

Day-by-Day Sprouting Progress... with Pictures!

Here's a pictorial view of the process of sprouting. I generally use a half-gallon jar for my sprouts. Simple and cheap. It makes enough for 2 hungry people for several days worth of delicious sprouts!

Day 1: Measure, clean junk out, and add sprouting seeds, beans, nuts, etc into your sprouting jar or tray.

Measure out your seeds/beans and glean the junk out of them. I usually do it while I'm slowly pouring them into the dry jar. It's rare to find junk in them any more, but it does happen.

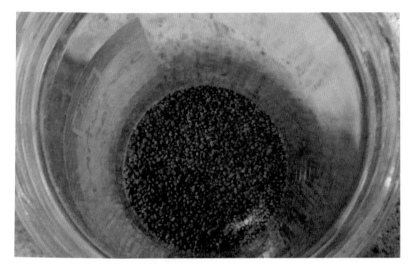

Not Much to See, Yet!

Still Day 1: Fill jar with plenty of water to begin soaking.

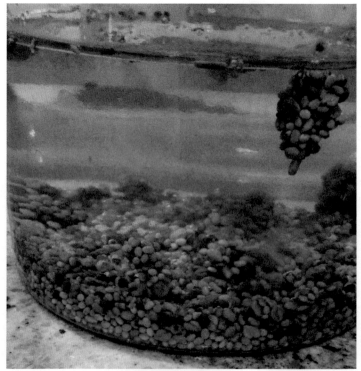

Just Add Water!

Some seeds will float and some will sink. Go figure. But, let them soak overnight. About 18 to 24 hours.

That's more than other books I've read about sprouting. But if I soak them longer, like this, then I don't have nearly the problem with them drying out later. Almost all problems I've had with batches, and there have been very few, had to do with them drying out. So, this extra soaking time really seems to give the sprouts a bit of water momentum, so to speak. It gives them enough soaked up water to carry them through my memory lapses or absences. The result is, more successful batches of fresh, homegrown sprouts make it to my tummy!

In the old system, if I missed a watering or two, I could lose a whole batch. This extra time soaking gives them *water momentum* to carry them through the dry spots.

Day 2: Drain, Rinse, Drain, Roll and Lay on Side!

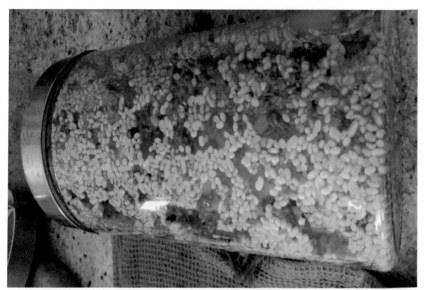

Drain, Rinse, Drain Again, Lay on Side, and Gently Roll to Spread Seeds Out!

Pretty cool looking, eh? Larger sprouts won't stick as well. No big deal. You can just be sure to turn the jar a couple of times a day. It keeps what residual water you might have in the jar circulating among the seeds. Extra time involved? Oh, about 2 seconds.

You'll do at least 2 rinse, drain, roll, and lay on side operations every day. So far, you've used up a minute and fourteen seconds in the first 2 days! Is that too much work, you, you counter-top farmers?

I didn't count the time I spend hunting for my measuring cup or other kitchen-based search and rescue operations (Like, "Where'd I put those sprouting seeds?") Granted, we all have days where we can't find anything and it seems to take forever. But it's easy to track it all if you keep it in a single shelf in the cupboard. Tah dah!

Day 3: Brings the Rinse and Repeat Process... and Budding Sprouts!

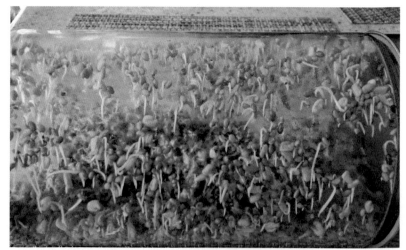

Day 3: Beginning to Look Like Sprouts!:

Day 3 brings another 14 seconds of rinse, drain, roll, and gently set down. Most sprouts begin to sprout on this day.

Here's where I begin to have problems with patience! They begin to look mighty tasty. Try to wait at least another day... two if you can stand it.

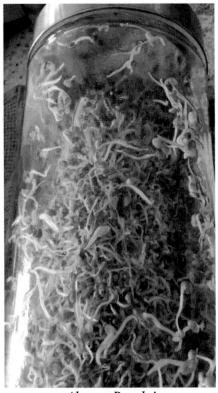

Almost Ready!

By the third day, you can eat most sprouts. Many can be eaten after the second day. Sometimes you run out of fresh sprouts, so you want to just grab some off the hoof. Go ahead.

Day 4: Shows Sprouts Growing and Bulking Up!

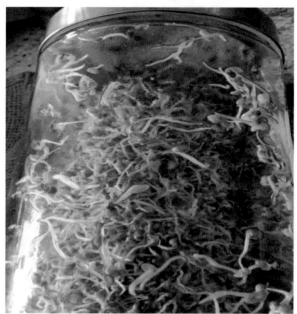

No Leaves Yet, Wait Another Day

The jar began with 1/3 cup of seeds 4 days ago. Now it's about 1/3 to ½ full of wonderful, healthy sprouts! By the end off the day, I'll begin to see sparse leaves forming and some greening. Generally I'll wait another day for seed sprouts. I want to get a large yield and lots of chlorophyll.

With larger sprouts like lentils, mung beans, and other beans, they can usually be eaten after 3 days. If you're cooking them in a soup, stew, or baking, that's fine. They are also good to snack on (Just pull out a pinch or two and pop them into your mouth!

Day 5: Brings More Bulk and More Green Leaves!

Spread the sprouts out on a tray, cookie sheet, or just on a clean counter top. Let them soak up some light and green up. Be sure to rinse and drain prior to setting them out to green up.

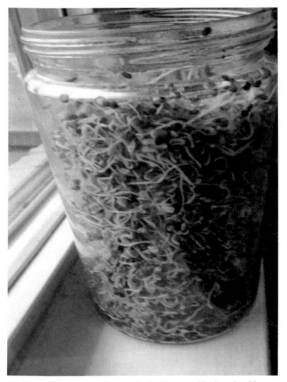

Day 5 Greening Up! Note all the hulls.

You'll get the knack in time and with repetition. Also, as you sprout more and more batches, you will begin to know when to start pilfering sprouts on the hoof (IE pulling out and using some sprouts while they are still in process). That's just fine and is actually a pretty common thing to do.

With smaller seeds, like alfalfa and the smaller seed mixes like what I've shown you here, I will sometimes let them stay out and actively sprouting (IE rinse, drain, and carefully set sideways on the counter.).

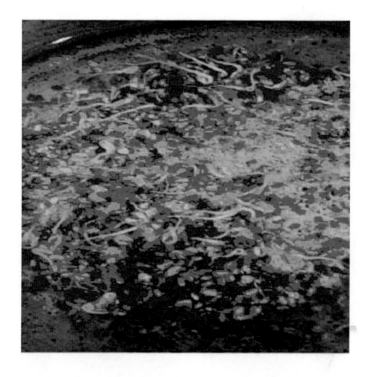

Day 5: Here you see the excess hulls!

Those last couple of extra days, I'm pulling sprouts out for each meal and for snacks. The interesting thing is that each day brings a re-fill! The sprouts continue to grow and replenish what I take out.

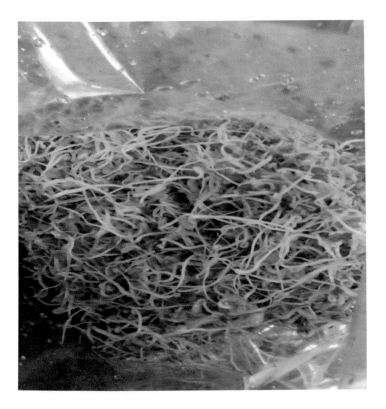

See how nice they look with NO hulls? I already have them in a bag for the fridge!

It's not a consistently uniform process, though. Each sprout has it's own maximum, optimal size. Beyond that they may begin to taste bitter or they may get tough and fibrous. No big deal. If they've gone too long, just pop them in your juicer with your other veggies. The bitterness, what little there is, is usually lost in the process of juicing.

Many of my readers have asked me what sprouts should look like during the process. I hope the pictures in this book help you get started.

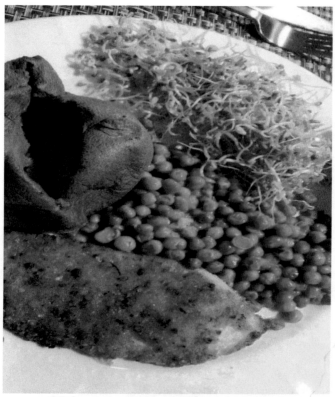

Fish, peas, sweet taters, and sprouts!
Mmmmmmmmmmmmmmmm, Let's Eat!

If you're doing the math, you probably already realized that it only takes about two-and-a-half minutes to grow a batch of sprouts in five-days!

When you read about how quick this process is, only taking about five minutes a week, you thought there's no way to do all that in such a small amount of time! Now you can see that it's really done in half the time!

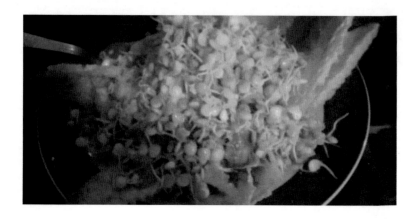

6: What I Sprout

I sprout for flavor, convenience, health and affordability. I sprout to participate in my own healthy food chain! I call it Self-Health!

Also, when I grow my own sprouts, I know how fresh, pure, and clean they are. I participated in their production. I know where they've been.

Store-bought pre-sprouted sprouts just never look very fresh to me and they don't seem to stay fresh very long. It's hard to know how far they traveled and how long they've been on the road before I buy them at the store.

That's a big part of why I keep a variety of dried beans and seeds on hand to keep a variety of sprouts harvesting in my kitchen on a constant, on-going basis. I usually vary each batch a bit. Once I might sprout lentils. Then, after I pull them out, I'll put some alfalfa in to sprout. Next I might sprout a mix of lentils and mung beans. Next maybe one of the sprouting mixes, like the Zesty Sprout mix from Now Foods (See Appendix).

In the winter I tend to grow more lentils and mung bean sprouts. I like them best of all in the many soups and stews I make in cold weather.

But I'm always making salads, so keep lots of smaller seeds sprouted, too, year-around. I usually keep 2 batches in some process of sprouting at any given time.

Sprouts are little nuggets of super nutrition. They contain all of the biochemicals necessary to produce an entire plant. You take a carb-loaded bunch of seeds, grains, or beans and turn them into the greatest nutritional source possible for pennies! And you do it on *your own kitchen counter,* simply and easily!

The following sprouts are not listed in any particular order. It's just the order that came to mind. It's also a reflection of what sprouts I make up the most of and the most often. I figure that what came to mind first were what were more important to my usual sprouting routine, so there you go.

Lentils

First on the list are lentils. I usually use what are generally called green lentils... although they look brown to me. You can get them at any grocery store, even Wal-Mart! Any more, I spring for organics at Whole Foods or Central Market or any of a bunch of natural markets. But still, occasionally, usually when I'm traveling in remote areas in my RV or sailboat, I'll just use the 88-cents-a-pound available-anywhere retail lentils. They all work!

In the past 3 years, I've only gotten one batch of beans that refused to sprout! Years ago, it was the rule. They were all sprayed or irradiated or somehow treated to prevent them from sprouting in storage. They put heaven-knows-what on them to give them longer shelf lives! No telling what that did for us when we ate them. But that's another book, later.

I think it's good to know that most all beans and seeds at most all stores now sprout just fine! That makes them so much more available to us all!

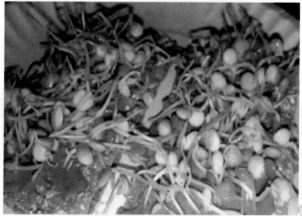

Lentils Make Tasty Sprouts!

Lentils are my favorite because they provide a ton of

wonderful food (AKA sprouts!) for pennies. They are also very hardy and seem to sprout well everywhere I've tried. I remember sprouting them in Baja, Mexico, in the Sea of Cortez, on my sailboat, when the temperature was around 112 degrees, dropping to 107 at night. Lentil sprouts never went sour or spoiled in that blazing heat and soaking humidity. Pretty much everything else I tried to sprout in those conditions failed nastily!

Lentils are very forgiving and have a mild flavor making them great for ANY application you think to try them in! Anything! And they keep well for a long time with or without refrigeration.

And by the way, if you're not using refrigeration, don't keep them in a plastic bag! Keep them in a colander or other well-ventilated container. If bugs are a problem, then you might consider making a fine screen mesh container to place over them or get one of those picnic screens that look like half-domes of mesh fabric over a small wire frame. They are great for placing over food to keep bugs off.

Alfalfa

I buy these in bulk (most recently, I bought a 3-pound bag of organic, non-GM alfalfa seeds for $18.00 on eBay with free shipping! See Appendix for details!). This will last me a couple of *years*... or maybe not. My last 2-pound bag lasted 2 years, but now, after writing and publishing this book, I keep sharing them with people who are interested in sprouting. I'm always happy to share what I have. Also, these days, I sprout more sprouts more often. So I go through them quicker these days. That's a good thing!

Sometimes you can find alfalfa seeds for sprouting at retail

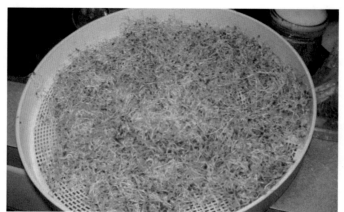

Alfalfa Sprouted in a DIY Re-Purposed Tray!

outlets at higher prices. But overall it's hard to find them due to the single-purpose nature of the seed. They are only used for sprouting. Lentils are mostly available and used for cooking, so they are more-readily available in retail outlets. Now Foods offers a pound bag (and smaller sizes, too!) of alfalfa seeds. Fresh and wonderful... and also budget-priced!

Alfalfa sprouts are wonderful for many reasons and a great addition to any meal, sandwich, or what-have-you. I generally grow a batch of alfalfa every second or third batch of sprouts.

I also mix alfalfa seeds to sprout seed mixes I buy. That way, it makes the more expensive mixes go further. Alfalfa have a mild flavor and a light texture, so they blend well with any other sprout. And they are just really nice to chew on.

Mung Beans

Lately I have been finding mung beans cheaper and cheaper. I found them at Whole Foods and Central Market the other day, (ORGANICS!) for only $2.50 a pound. A couple of days later I found the same organics at the another store for $2.17! I think people are starting to buy more of them, for cooking and sprouting, so prices are coming down!

A pound of mung beans goes a long way! I frequently sprout

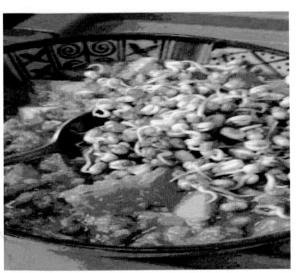

them 50/50 with lentils in a mix. They have a nice, mild flavor and heavy yields! Every third or fourth batch, I'll make a pure batch of just mung beans. Mmmmm, good!

Wheat

I grow wheat grass for juicing, but don't have a good system down, yet. I grow the wheat grass in dirt and sometimes in sprouting trays!

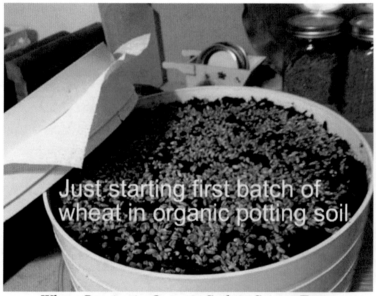

Wheat Berries in Organic Soil, in Sprout Tray

But for sprouting, wheat berries, are just plain wonderful! Follow the process I showed you for sprouting, but harvest them when they get about 1/4" to 3/4" long. In this case, don't "green them up."

They are so very sweet, it's just amazing. Makes a nice, sweet, and nutty-tasting snack! Grind them up and add them to your baking recipes. Put them whole in soups, on salads, in sandwiches. And set out a bowl of them for snacking!

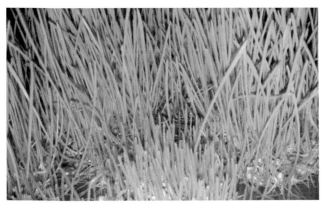

Greened Up, Ready to Juice!

Wheat is one of the cheapest sprouts you can buy. I did some research a while back about gluten content in wheat sprouts. Most of the info I found said that wheat sprouts contain gluten. However, if you plant or sprout wheat berries and cut the grass when it's about 6" long, it gets juiced and has NO gluten in it. So if you have some gluten intolerance, stick with that most wonderful of green juices, wheat grass juice!

Chickpeas (Garbanzo Beans)

Occasionally I'll sprout some chickpeas. I use them in bigger meals like chunky veggie soup or on salads. They make a nice snack food for company, you know, "regular folks," people who don't know about sprouts and would normally be eating salted, roasted, MSG-ed peanuts.

You see garbanzo beans sprouted in many salad bars. Frequently they've been soaked in vinegar, too. The sprouts tend to be shorter. I keep mine fairly short, too, around 1/4" to 1/2".

I'll harvest Garbanzos when they have a shaft about a quarter to half an inch long. Why? It seems that these beans have a greater propensity than others to spoil when sprouting. They get what I call, "The Slime Goin' On!" When I get to hankerin' for sprouted chick peas, I'll be sure to rinse them lots more (4 times a day or more!), drain them well, and keep a close eye on them. The extra effort is well rewarded with a delicious sprout!

In recipes calling for cooked chickpeas or ground chickpeas, the sprouts add more nutrition and better flavor, says Jim B!

Sunflower

I love (*Absolutely* LOVE!) the flavor and texture of sunflower seed sprouts. They are soooooo gooood! I grow them differently than other sprouts, though.

For nice long straight sprout shafts, I grow them in about an inch of organic soil. I plant raw, in the shell, sunflower seeds (Be sure to soak them overnight, first!). I prefer to let them grow as tall as they want, only cutting them off above the soil level when they just begin to show second set of leaves coming.

You have to wash them / rinse them more so than other sprouts to get the organic soil off of them. But you only have to do that once, when you harvest them.

If I'm sprouting them in a jar, I use hulled sunflower seeds, always organic. Before soaking them, I spread them out on a plate and cull out the broken seeds. The broken seeds are more likely to just turn to mush when you try to sprout them. So get them out before you get started. Just work with whole, well-formed seeds.

Sunflower seed sprouts tend to grow more curly in the jar or tray, IE. without soil. I usually harvest them earlier, too as the "root" part gets to tasting too bitter for my preference and can begin to detract from the wonderful flavor of sunflower seed sprouts.

The allure of sunflower seed sprouts, for me, is the wonderful textures they share when I chew them up and also the complex flavors they impart. Yep, my favorites!

Peanuts

Yes, I said peanuts! Get a bag of *raw* peanuts. Neither roasted nor baked nor with any additives. Just raw peanuts. Most stores sell them nowadays, pretty cheap, too. I think even Wal-Mart sells a pound bag of raw peanuts for about 2 bucks, but you have to shell them before you sprout them. It's fairly labor-intensive that way. And a lot of the peanuts get mysteriously eaten during the process.

More and more, I have been finding raw, shelled peanuts at larger grocers, natural food stores, and online. The online route tends to be the more expensive route in this case, as the shipping cost per seed is high due to the bigger-sized "seeds" that peanuts are.

My sprouting process for peanuts is a bit different. Simply soak them 18 to 24 hours like any other sprouts. Rinse them and bag them. Serve them as a snack.

Sometimes I'll keep them soaking, changing the water each day, for 2 days.

The sprouted peanut is MUCH more digestible for me and a better food value than a raw peanut or one that's been baked, broiled, boiled, roasted, or fried. It doesn't even taste like a peanut any more! Peanut sprouts are crunchy and taste more like water chestnuts.

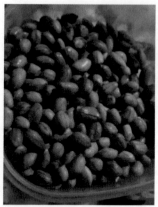

Raw Peanuts Ready to Sprout!

You can try to follow the basic sprouting procedure with them. I don't think they taste as good once they get an inch or more in sprout length. But you might enjoy them. And they'll be more nutritionally potent.

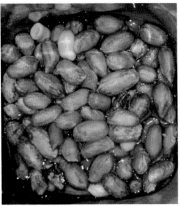

After 24 Hours of Soaking,, Ready to Enjoy!

Also, once you've tried sprouted peanuts the way I've just told you about, you won't be able to wait for them to sprout any bigger before you start eating them! They're *that* good!

Peanuts generally swell up to about twice their original size, too. Put out a bowl of them on card night and watch people eat them up. Don't tell them what they are eating until they ask for more. They'll be amazed and so will you!

Black-Eyed Peas

Black-eyed peas are my favorite tasting sprouts (Have you noticed how many sprouts are my *favorite* sprouts? I like them all so very much!). I don't sprout black-eyed peas as much as I'd like to. They're best grown in cooler seasons as I'll explain below.

I really enjoy the sprouting process for black-eyed peas. It brings the beans back to life, greening them up and adding a nice young plant shoot, too. The flavor is wonderfully nutty. If you have ever eaten fresh-picked black-eyed peas, you know the flavor!

I don't sprout them much because they are very quick to go slimy on me. In warmer weather, especially in the tropics, they'll go slimy in a day. When it's really hot, it's really hard to get them to sprout all the way. That is, of course, if you don't have air conditioning!

In the winter I try to get a few batches done and never regret it. They are so delicious.

It's important to rinse them more often than other sprouts. The extra effort will be rewarded.

Almonds

You can sprout raw almonds just the same as with peanuts. They make great snacks and are great for use in making nut milks and butters!

A friend of mine had a couple of very nice looking almond trees he had started from raw almonds. They started as sprouts, but got too big to eat... so he planted them! They were lovely plants and were a great way to re-purpose almond sprouts.

Beans

You can sprout just about any dried beans. Whenever possible, be sure to get organics. Better beans make better sprouts. Chemical-laden beans make chemical-laden sprouts. Your choice.

If they fail to sprout after a few days, you can be sure they've either been irradiated or sprayed with some nasty chemical to keep them from sprouting. It could also be that they are so old they're germ is dead.

If you find some type you really like, let me know and tell me how you did it. I'll include it in this book and give you heaps of praise and notoriety!

Other Sprouts You Can Try

Most of the sprouts in this category are things I sprouted in "mixes" I've bought. Some are occasional sprouts that I'll sprout up now and again. Some are fine, sprouted individually. Others are best when blended to cut down on strong flavors. Radishes and dill are that way for me. I prefer to sprout them in a mix to diffuse the strong flavor a bit.

Other sprouts were sprouted in mixes as they were pretty pricey per pound and only affordable when I bought a few ounces at a time. To help them go further, I blended them with other, more affordable seeds. I also think it's good to blend similarly-sized seeds for sprouting to give you a broader mix of nutrients to feed your one-hundred-plus billion cells!

Try them all for yourself and see what rewarding results you get. Share that info with me and I'll include your comments in my next edition and give you heaps of praise for your contribution!

Other sprouts I've had success with include:

- ✓ Anise
- ✓ Barley
- ✓ Broccoli
- ✓ Buckwheat
- ✓ Chia (With or without a terra cotta puppy!)
- ✓ Clover
- ✓ Cress
- ✓ Fenugreek
- ✓ Flax
- ✓ Kale
- ✓ Pea
- ✓ Radish
- ✓ Soybeans

Sprouting Mixes

I started buying bulk mixes of sprouts off the internet last year. It lets me try different sprouting seeds in a blended way. How wonderful can it get? The sprouting mixes I've tried (some with up to six different seeds!) are amazing! They give an explosion of flavors and textures when I pop them in my mouth.

As with any sprouts, I put them on everything! Soups, salads, sandwiches, main courses, and just eat them plain as a snack!

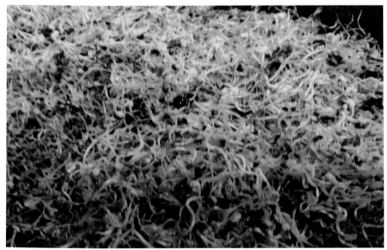

Sprout Mix with Clover, Radish, and Fenugreek

Some sprouts, like dill and radishes are a bit potent to the taste buds. By blending them in a mix, I get the great aromas and flavors, but don't get overwhelmed by them!

Since I buy my alfalfa seeds cheap in 2 to 3 pound bulk lots, I'll mix them with my pricey mixes to make the pricier mixes go further.

It's all so good!

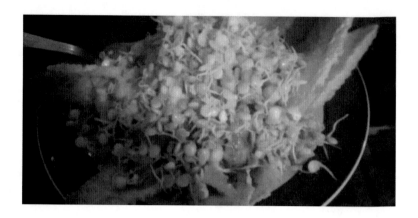

7: Types of Sprouters and DIY Sprouters!

It seems that every week somebody's coming up with another way to sprout sprouts! Some clever person has developed a travel sprouter for sprouting small amounts of sprouts in your suitcase, on the road! Too cool!

Here are some of the more common sprouting methods for you to look at.

Sprouting Trays

Sprouting trays are just that, trays. You can buy them as single trays and you can also find them in stackable trays that allow you to grow three or four (or more!) different sprouts at one time on your counter top without taking up too much counter space. They are finely grooved on the bottom floor of the trays to keep sprouting seeds out of standing water. The seeds can draw the water up into themselves via surface-tension action.

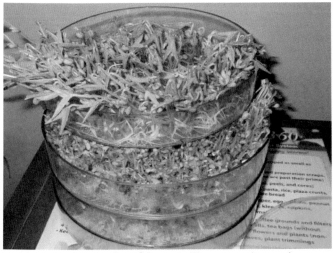

An Example of Sprout Trays in Action!

You can find a great variety of sizes and numbers of trays on the internet shopping sites. Shop around for what seems best for you and go for the best deal. With several stackable trays, you can sprout several different types of sprouts in a vertical stack, saving space. It's great for people with too many things vying for counter top space.

Re-Purposed Food Dehydrator Trays

Here's a cheap alternative to pricey sprouting trays! I've bought large numbers of stackable trays at yard sales for next to nothing. They were originally used in food dehydrators. I've gotten ten to twenty trays for a buck or two. They work great for the larger sprouting seeds, grains, nuts, and beans. It's an example of recycling and re-purposing at its best. It also allows me to be generous with people curious about sprouting. I can afford to share a couple of sprouting trays with them to help get them started.

Finding Used Sprouting Trays!

I've occasionally found real sprouting tray sets at yard sales, auctions, and thrift stores. They are much cheaper in those venues. For some reason, twenty cents worth of plastic costs twenty bucks when they press it into a sprouting tray. I do not like being taken advantage of when I'm only trying to eat healthy nutritious food. My desire for healthy food doesn't make me any less savvy a shopper, though. Pay a fare price, but don't pay too much for sprouting trays, because, after all, they're just plastic.

Any more, I sprout with glass jars just to be sure I'm not introducing any toxic chemistry from the plastics involved in trays. It's my own *thing* from being lied to by the plastics industry my whole life. I have been trying to phase myself out of plastics around my food. It may be a futile effort, but at least I'm trying to do better for myself.

Sprouting Bags

Sprouting bags are mesh bags you can buy to sprout in. I'm not so hot on them as they need a clean plate to sit on so as not to mess up the counter top or a hook to hang on with a drip pan below. Another reason they need to be kept on a plate is to keep them from soaking up any stray germs or chemistry from the counter top.

As they age, sprouting bags tend to stain from the tannins in the seeds you are sprouting.

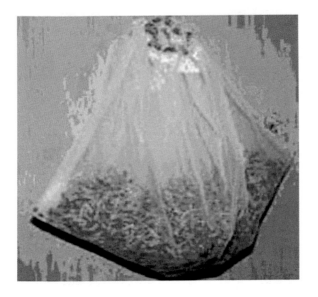

Example of a Sprouting Bag!

If the fabric mesh is too big, roots take hold and make it hard to get the bags cleaned when you are done.

Make Your Own Sprouting Bags

Got a sewing machine? You can buy the fabric and make your own sprouting bags for next to nothing! Send me some and I'll try them. If they work, I'll include a link to you in my next edition and say wonderful things about you!

Sprouting Jars

Now Foods sells a great ½ gallon jar with a stainless steel screen! You can pay more for them online, about nine to twelve bucks. But at local natural food stores, I've gotten them for just under five bucks to just under six bucks!

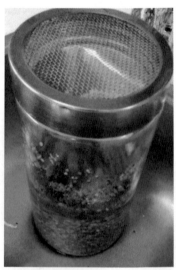

Read about them and find a retailer near you who sells them. Now Foods has a web site that lets you stick your zip code in and find nearby retailers who sell them. It makes it easy to get a great sprout system up and running for not much money.

Example of a Commercial Sprouting Jar!

Those big jars make great gifts for newbies! I fill them with a half dozen little zip bags of different seeds, beans, and nuts for people to get started with. Of course, that's why I wrote this little booklet, too. I wrote it to toss into the jar to show them how to get started sprouting.

You'll find more info at Now Foods

http://www.nowfoods.com/Sprouting-Jar.htm

These jars are nice looking, have a stainless steel lid and screen, and make about a half a gallon of sprouts. It's a great way to get started sprouting. BTW Now Foods did not solicit my recommendation. I just really like their sprouting jar and their sprouting seeds, too.

After that, there are only those cheap-o plastic sprouting jar lids of unknown toxicity that are available for much more money online! I've seen individual lids selling online for as much as $8 but never less than about 4 dollars. Then you have to get a jar... which is a simple matter as they are made for standard canning jars.

The Now Foods sprouting jars are a great value, I think! You get a great screen, lid, and jar... all in one for not much money. And they're usually available locally! Another plus to that is that when you buy your jar, you can pick up a small assortment of sprouting seeds and beans to get started with.

Again, if you find something better, please spread the word. We sprouters need to stick together!

Another great alternative, if you can find them or make them, is to get stainless steel screen mesh cut to fit the lids to canning jars. You can get a case of quart or half-gallon canning jars, with lids, for about ten to twelve bucks. Use the screens with them and you've got an army of sprouting jars! Sometimes you can find the mesh screens, pre-cut to fit the canning jars, on eBay or Amazon.

Sprouting in Dirt

I've never done well sprouting sunflower seeds. I can get a batch done, but they never look as nice as they do when I've seen them at farmers markets. When I sprout them in a jar or on a tray, they come out looking all twisted up. But they still taste great!

Now and again, I'll plant them in an inch or two of organic potting soil and let them sprout and grow up to about 3" - 4" tall where they are just beginning to show their second leaves. Then I can just cut the amount I want and trim off more as needed. Mmmmm good... and great texture!!!

I also sprout wheat seeds in dirt to get nice uniform wheat grass for juicing!

It takes six days for wheat to sprout and grow to about 6" high for juicing. I usually plant enough to give me several days' worth of grass for juicing. Then, every 3 days I start another dirt farm pot of wheat to keep the process going.

For general sprouting purposes, however, I sprout wheat like any other sprout... dirt-less. Sprouted wheat is sweet and crunchy and has an almost nutty flavor!

You can grow dirt-types of sprouts in a windowsill or on your kitchen counter, too!

All you need is a good pot, some organic potting soil, and some wheat berries to grow.

DIY Sprouting Set-Ups

Canning jars! That's the answer for the DIY sprouter! Use the canning jar with the 2-part lid. I use either the 1-quart or half-gallon size jars (mostly I rely on the half gallon jars to give me the sprout yields I want!). I think it's better to use the wider mouth jars, by the way.

Remove the solid insert from the 2-part lid assembly. Take the open lid-ring and cut a piece of cheesecloth or fiberglass screen material to use for the insert on the lid.

These do-it-yourself sprouting jars are wonderful and easy to use. Did I mention that they are also about as inexpensive a way to sprout as you can devise?

Also, keep an eye out at yard sales and thrift stores for old food dehydrator trays. They make great sprouters. See below: One of the over 20 trays I bought at a yard sale for nine bucks, years ago, and still use today!

The El Cheapo Method!

If you're really cheap, like me, and want to get started without spending any money buying a sprouting jar or tray setup, just wash up an old mayo jar, jelly jar, or drinking water glass. Using larger beans like lentils, you can begin growing sprouts.

When you get done soaking and need to drain the jar, just put your hand over the opening and let your fingers sieve the water out and keep the beans in. You can then cover the opening with a paper towel or clean dishtowel to keep the bugs out and let the air flow in!

Simple, cheap, easy, and instant. Your Jim-B-DIY-Sprouter!

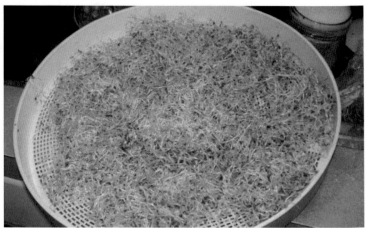

Tray Sprouter DIY from Old Dehydrator Trays!

Faster, Better, Gimmick Sprouters

I keep seeing new-fangled sprouters for sale on eBay, Amazon, and around the internet. So far I've managed to resist buying any of them. Many of them cost too much money for the benefits they promise.

Sprouting is such a simple, low-tech way to produce the best food on the planet that I don't see why anyone would want to waste money on gimmicks that don't really add to the process?

My Sprouter Preference (And "Why!")

Overall, I prefer to use glass jars for sprouting. The principle reason is that glass has less chance of introducing chemical pollution to the sprouting process. Glass jars are easier to keep clean, too. Plastics, for all they have infiltrated our lives, still bring the risk of toxic chemistry. I've had enough of that for this lifetime!

Lately, I have been hearing about "new-fangled" plastics that don't possess bad chemistry. In years past, I also read about "new-fangled" plastics that were said to alleviate bad chemistry. But they ended up bringing us even worse chemistry in the process. So, I'll wait a long time before I present yet another toxic risk to my poor old wretched self or to you, my friends.

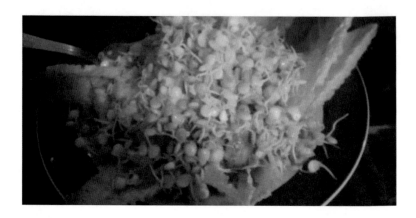

8: Where to Get Seeds for Sprouting!

No secrets here. Sprouting seeds, beans, nuts and grains are available all over the place. You just have to look around with your sprouter's eyes.

Most natural food stores have bulk products. Lentils, mung beans, adzuki beans, etc are easy to find in bulk. Same with the basic sprouting grains and nuts When you get grains, make sure they are whole grains and not bleached, rolled, cut, or roasted. Same with nuts. You always want to get "raw" nuts and seeds.

The first time you try a new thing to sprout or the first time you buy an old standby from a new source, be sure to get just enough for one or two batches. That way, if they turn out to be poor producers or fail altogether, you won't be out much money.

Any more, organics are not much more costly than non-organics. Get organics! If you're one of the old timers who hold onto the thought that there is no difference between organics and non-organics (And I know you're out there!)... get over it... NOW! There is such a huge difference, the life you save may be your own!

If you are out in the boonies and can only find non-organics, go for it. It's better to eat healthy sprouts whatever way you can find them. Most supermarkets still sell a pound of lentils for about a buck. That will make up about a half dozen ½-gallons of fresh sprouts!

Most all supermarkets still have a small shelf of dried beans. Any more you can find sproutable beans there! For the past few years, all of the beans I've bought from traditional grocers have sprouted just fine. I think they finally quit spraying or irradiating them prior to packaging. Hurray!

Some natural food markets are making a larger variety of seeds available for sprouting. I can find alfalfa seeds, broccoli seeds, and lots of different seeds at local natural grocers and health food stores.

With Amazon Prime membership, you can get free 2nd day air shipping on your sprouting seeds making mail order more affordable!

I have been buying bulk sprouting seeds on eBay and at Amazon online for the past several years. Just a few months ago, I bought 3 pounds of organic, non-GM, alfalfa seeds on eBay for $18 (with free shipping). That'll last me a year or more, even though I give away baggies of them all the time for new sprouters to try.

I found bulk (1 pound bags) of nice sprout mixes, too, online at eBay and Amazon. It's a simple search online. Search for keywords SPROUT SEEDS.

Online, search for keywords SPROUT SEEDS

One mix I bought was a mix of radish seeds and kale. A pound was about 22 bucks I also got a mix of 6 seeds for about 25 bucks. Those types of mixed sprouts are really fun to grow and eat! For that pound of smaller seeds, I'll probably get 20 half-gallon yields of wonderful sprout mixes!

To save some money on the process, I mix my higher-priced sprout mixes with alfalfa, which only costs me about 6 bucks a pound. The resultant mix is just fine and maybe even more fun to eat.

Never, absolutely never, buy seeds for sprouting that have been especially prepared for planting in traditional agriculture! Those planting seeds are generally coated with all sorts of wicked chemistry that can be poisonous! When you buy beans, grains, and seeds labeled for human consumption, you are safe! Read labels closely if you are looking at organic *planting* seeds, too! Make sure they are safe to eat.

Here's another unsolicited plug for Now Foods! They offer their Zesty Sprouting Mix, locally, for about six bucks a pound! They also sell Alfalfa seeds for sprouting locally for the same price! They also offer smaller amounts of broccoli seeds for sprouting. That company really seems to be in the business of supporting healthy food, diet, and lifestyles! Nobody does that better... says me.

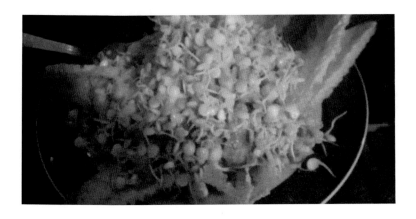

9: Some Notes about Sprouting!

Message from a New Sprouter, Grace

My friend, Grace, called from New Jersey. She was a novice sprouter and said the white beans she was trying to sprout just turned into a smelly, gooey, nasty mess. She'd tried it 3 times. It was sad because this was Grace's first time to try sprouting!

I told her the beans were probably just bad beans for sprouting. Many "regular" grocery stores stock dried beans that are sprayed with chemicals or irradiated to keep them from sprouting if they get some moisture into the bags (although they are doing that less and less!). It's done to improve the shelf life of the product. It's a measure to protect their bottom line... while degrading your own health in the process.

Also, I told Grace, the beans could just be so very old, they are no longer viable. She tossed them and went and got some organic beans and is now a happy sprouter, busy sprouting everything she can get her hands on! She's also busy finding new converts to the world of wonderful, healthy sprouts!

5-Star Book Reviews: Changing Lives!

This Book Is Changing Lives! Not just mine, either. When I began sharing my story with friends, they invariably asked me more and more questions. Once I got the book done, I ran it past my friends and began to see and hear stories of profound personal growth and change!

This is not a book to simply read. It's a book you must experience! It will change your life!

Here's an example of how this book is changing lives! This person relates how my experience at reversing my problems motivated her to do the same…

BySister Mary Debrechton October 24, 2015

Format: PaperbackVerified Purchase

"I found the book very helpful in guiding me to venture into sprouting. His reasons for sprouting and his results were all I needed to get started. Now that I am into sprouting, I wouldn't be without my sprouts every day. No work

involved really. Try it. You will like it! One of the best
health projects you could ever take up."

Here's what my dear friend of 30 years, Kate Quimby, had to
say when she'd read the book. She gave 5-Star Feedback for the
book, Sprouting: The Beginners Guide to Growing Sprouts! on
Amazon.com:

> ***A basic practical sprouting book from an***
> ***inspired, enlightened author with a good heart!***
>
> *By Kate Quimby on March 29, 2015*
>
> ***Verified Purchase***
>
> *I know this author, not a relative but a friend*
> *from afar, and this guy is genuine. If I was*
> *stranded on a desert island, I would choose him*
> *if I could only have one other person. Anything*
> *he writes is from the heart and you can depend*
> *on it. He's inspired me to start sprouting again*
> *and he's not paying me to write this! Enjoy!*

I emailed a big thanks to Kate, who lives over 1100 miles from
me, to thank her for her very nice feedback. What follows is the
email I got in return...

> *"… Right now I am eating a plate of eggs, onion,*
> *small peppers, avocado, and HOME GROWN*
> *SPROUTS! Thanks to you.*
>
> *Didn't want to embarrass you with the review*
> *but when I thought about it a while and realized*
> *that the people who would be interested in your*

book would enjoy this review and it could excite others to get to know this "enlightened author"!

I'm overwhelmed with the reviews this book is getting. There are millions of us, starved for real nutrition and health in a country overstocked with devitalized food and bad information.

I knew how my life had been changed, but seeing and hearing from others is another thing altogether. It's with gratitude that I tell my tale about sprouts!

Warm Weather / Cool Weather Sprouting

In warmer weather, rinse the sprouts more often and drain longer (...about 5 to 6 seconds longer). Cooler weather can let you get by with 2 rinses a day. If you ever notice some sliminess, rinse them more than usual. If the sliminess returns, the batch may have gone bad. NEVER eat slimy sprouts! But try to rinse at least 2 or 3 times a day to insure the best yield possible.

If you keep your sprouts in a cooler environment, rinse a couple of times a day, they should always work out fine for you.

Sprouting New Things

If you get curious about sprouting something new, just look it up on the internet. Be sure to read several articles on the subject before you get started. I've often found that opinions about how to sprout different things can vary widely and wildly. A good example is when I wanted to try to sprout peanuts. I finally tried it using a little information from several articles and my own intuition.

Fabulous results!

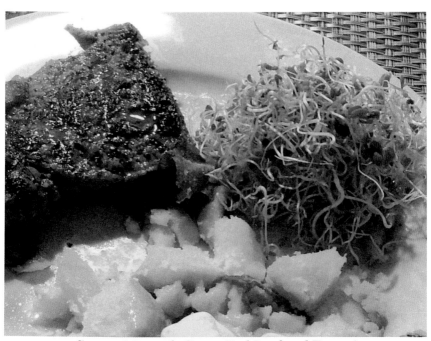

Sprout Mix with Grass-Fed Beef and Taters!

Sprouting Rice

I've heard that sprouting rice is really wonderful. I don't have first hand experience, yet. As of this writing, I've only tried sprouting rice one time. It didn't work. Although it was organic whole grain rice, it just slowly turned to mush. I'll try again another day. If you've had luck with rice, let me know so I can pass the info on!

Why This Book Doesn't...

Tell You How To Sprout Everything!

There are lots of sprouting sites on the internet. They have lists of jillions of types of sprouts and how to sprout them. That's why I don't have an anthological list of sprouts in my book. This book is intended to give you a simple, reproducible method of sprouting that can be adapted to most everything you might want to sprout.

The second goal is to help you keep sprouting on an ongoing basis to insure you always have plenty of fresh, home-grown sprouts to eat, every day!

Those 2 concepts, when combined and practiced will make you an independent self-health / self-help expert for a lifetime of better you and wonderful sprouts.

So, rather than making you dependent on my book or my site, I'm trying to give you the skills you need to do this yourself on an ongoing basis.

Let's all get better!

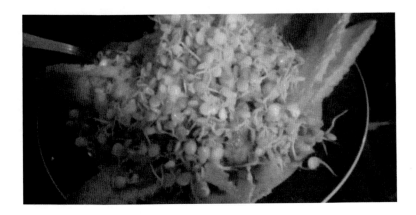

10: Serving Sprouts!

Now you're a *sprouter!* What's next? Ya gotta eat them, that's what's next! As exciting a picture as I paint about the sprouting process, the best is yet to come! There's an endless variety of ways to eat sprouts, incorporate sprouts into dishes, and include them in every meal!

This book is chock full of lovely pictures of sprouts ready to eat in wonderful ways. When you go to my website, www.BeginnersGuideToSprouting.com, you'll see more pictures of sprouts presented at various meals, ready to go. These aren't staged pictures shot by a professional, either. As I got healthier and happier about my changes for the better, at some point I decided to take pictures of the meals I was making. I was sure it would be better to show people than trying to describe them. And, for once, I was right. People just love the pictures of the colorful, healthy meals I prepare. When I simply described them without pictures, the more frequent response was "eeeeeuuuuwwwwww."

That response was because so many of my friends ate like I used to. So describing a plant-based dinner, lunch, breakfast, or snack sounded awful to them. But the pictures spoke volumes about the wonderful food prepared so delightfully! I'd post those pictures on my personal Facebook page, and later, on the Facebook page devoted to this book. Go to www.Facebook.com and search for "Sprouting: The Beginners Guide to Growing Sprouts" or simply enter the URL, *https://www.facebook.com/pages/Sprouting-The-Beginners-Guide-to-Growing-Sprouts/644738185672813*

It turns out that pictures draw us all in to good, healthy food because, I think, it just looks wonderful. It says, "Eat me, I'm amazing!" Or, to borrow an old sales slogan from the meat-eating world, "The sizzle sells the steak!" In this case, the sprouts!

Eat Sprouts All By Themselves!

The simplest way to eat sprouts is to just grab a pinch between your thumb and forefinger and pop them in your mouth, raw, alone, unseasoned, and wonderful. When I'm harvesting sprouts from the sprouting jar to the plastic bag, I always grab a few bites. They haven't greened up yet, but they are already wonderful!

Once the sprouts are greened up and in the fridge, I can grab a pinch of them anytime through the day when a snack is in order. An old friend's only comment about that is, "Tastes like dirt!" I'm not sure he eats much beyond fast food. I've noticed people who don't eat raw veggies in any quantities seem to possess the most contempt prior to investigation regarding sprouts. They are conditioned to immediate gratification on some level not related to real food. I used to be that way. "Lettuce?" "By itself?" "Me?" "You crazy!"

Set Sprouts on the Table at EVERY Meal!

Start with baby steps. Just begin to set them out on the table at every meal. EVERY MEAL! They might just sit there looking at you. But if you have them out, you might try adding some to something. This is a non-recipe approach to eating sprouts.

Put a dollop of sprouts on your meat, your potatoes, your veggies, your salad. Put a dollop on the side of your plate and pick some sprouts up with your fork and then pick up a bit of something from your plate. How does that taste? How does it feel in your mouth? How does it look? If you begin to experiment, you'll begin to find what you like and don't like sprouts on.

Try it more than once. Also, repeat the personal taste experiment with each new and different batch of sprouts. Different sprouts go differently with different foods. When I first got ahold of NOW FOODS Zesty Sprouting Mix I didn't think it would go well with other foods, what with it being *zesty* and all. Who knew? I loved it. It enhanced steaks, fish, and other meats, especially grilled meats! It livened up my salads! It gave a life worth living to sandwiches! It went well with eggs for breakfast. By keeping an open mind and trying them on all sorts of different foods, I discovered that sprouts really do go well with everything.

If you are reading this book for the first time and are new to sprouting, you're in for a treat! The voyage of discovery is wonderful. I wish you wonderful lovely meals made so much better with sprouts!

Stews, soups, and stir-fries! Steaks, salads, and shish kabobs. Sandwiches, breads, and on anything cooked or raw.

Soups and Stews, Before and After!

Sometimes I cook my soups and stews with larger sprouts, like lentils, mung beans, and black-eyed peas. They can cook down a bit and add some body to the concoction. Then, when I serve it up, I will put finer sprouts on top, like alfalfa, clover, or that Zesty sprout mix. They mix in well and add a savory crunch to soups and stews.

Sandwiches!

Sandwiches. I haven't tried sprouts on peanut butter... *yet*. But I say, *yet*, because at some point I'm gonna make me a peanut butter sandwich and will be trying sprouts on it. I'll let ya know what I think.

Meanwhile, sprouts can be added to just about any sandwich simply enough. Just like you'd put lettuce on a sandwich, a nice layer of sprouts adds to the presentation, curb appeal, of the sandwich, as well as adding to the flavors and textures and overall healthiness of the thing. I use whatever sprouts I have around and have never gotten anything but great results.

Going to Subway or other sandwich shop? Take along a zip bag of sprouts and add them to your sandwich. Heck, if you're still eating at McDonald's and the like, take sprouts with you to health-up your sandwiches!

Sandwiches I've made using sprouts include (this list is only limited by my poor memory): egg salad, tofu salad, turkey, chicken, chicken salad, fried-egg, grilled cheese, cheese, cucumber, sautéed fish, shrimp, ham, olive loaf, veggie burger, hamburger, black-bean paste, curried tofu, and on and on. If it's a sandwich, it deserves sprouts. Try it, you'll see.

Notes About Veggie Burgers!

Veggie burgers and veggie loafs are something that I fix up a lot. I use a slow-masticating juicer to make my fresh veggie juices (and YES, I always put a bunch of fresh sprouts in my juices!). I run the fiber through the juicer a second time to pull out more nutrients and juice. When I get done, there's always leftover fiber just for my imagination to utilize!

I usually do one of three things with it: make up veggie burgers, make up a veggie loaf, or make up a veggie soup stock. When veggie burgers or loaves are on the menu, I always add plenty of sprouts to the mix. It helps hold them together and gives them a nice flavor. It seems to work well with any sprouts I have on hand. See what you think.

Casseroles

Pretty much any casseroles I make up are gonna get some sprouts in them, either in the beginning or on top when served!

Baking!

I like various bean sprouts for baking: lentil, mung, and black-pea. I've sprouted wheat berries and added them to my bread machine. They came out fine. But I don't use the bread machine any more. I really don't each much bread. Not sure why. I'd guess it's because I mostly eat veggies and raw foods.

Second most difficult arena is breakfast!

Sprouts for breakfast? Really? Yes. Start slow. I started with eggs. I'd put a dollop of sprouts on the side of my plate. They looked nice there and gave more color to the meal... as those sort of egg-based breakfasts can be fairly monochromatic.

I tried a few sprouts on my fork and then grabbing some egg. Tasted great and felt great in my mouth! If the yolk was runny, all the better! Gave some crunch and felt great in my mouth. Tasted wonderful, too. Who knew?

Next came oatmeal! "Oatmeal?" I see that look of OMG in your mind! Try it, with a slight disclaimer. I eat my oatmeal without sugars or milks. I like it with butter and some garlic. Sometimes I add a bit of finely shredded cheese to my oatmeal and stir it in. Mmmm good. Try it before you knock it.

So, upon that base of perspective toward my oatmeal eating, I put some sprouts on top of a bowl of oatmeal. It was great! I tried stirring it in to blend it. With the smaller sprouts, they get a bit limp, but it's not a bad effect. I prefer them crispy, though, so usually put them on the side. You'll notice that in my breakfast pictures. I generally put them on the side.

Grits? Y'all eat grits? I do. Same way as I like my oatmeal. Might even add some curry or cumin to it! Sprouts go great with it.

Back to eggs. Omelets? Inside or on top, sprouts make any egg dish gourmet looking, more delicious, and more inviting. Ya just gotta try it. Sometimes I'll stir-fry some sprouts or put them inside an omelet, raw. It truly is "all good."

Frittatas? Mmmm good. Cooking them with sprouts or donning sprouts on top, way, you are in for a treat.

I even put fresh sprouts on top of my French toast, twice so far! It was wonderful, truly delightful. Go figure. I just thought I'd try. But the sprouts crunched and took on the flavors of the French toast and the pure maple surple. It worked! I had been sprouting for several years before I tried that, so I understand if you don't want to jump right in and try them that way. I have posted pictures to the Facebook page and the website, www.BeginnersGuideToSprouting.com, just to show you it can be done.

Most Difficult Arena for Sprouts: Desserts!

I've got nothing for you here. I don't eat traditional desserts any more. Not sure what to tell you. I do occasionally make fruit sorbet with frozen fruits and my slow-masticating juicer. I thought about adding sprouts to the sorbets, but couldn't bring myself to it.

I eat pretty healthy nowadays and haven't put much effort into making healthy alternatives to traditional desserts. If you do, let me know how it works out for you. I'd love to share it with everyone... and maybe even try it myself.

Wrapping It Up!

I prepare and/or cook most all of my own meals nowadays. It takes less time for me to prep a great healthy meal than it takes to drive down to a fast food joint, order, and wait in line for the devitalized food to be delivered to my car. The rewards for choosing to eat a healthy diet are beyond belief.

And, counting the gasoline used up and money spent on junk food, healthy food costs so much less! If you could figure it out at the rate of *Dollars / Ounce of Vital Food*, it would come out that healthy food is dirt cheap, and sprouts, as you now know, are dirtlessly cheap! Once again, who knew?

So I can make all sorts of great foods for myself in my own kitchen and I always have a good supply of fresh, homegrown sprouts on hand to augment each meal. Start with a pinch of sprouts out of the jar and plop them in your mouth. Do that and build on it as I've described here.

Don't have the time? Yes you do. How long does it take to grow a batch of sprouts? 5 minutes over 4 or 5 days! How long does it take to plop a pinch of sprouts in your mouth and chew them up? Seconds. No time for that? Remember, that's where you start. As the days roll forward, as you learn and grow, you'll wonder where all the extra time in each day has come from. Honest. Your own vital energy will return with a renewed vigor!

Congratulations, you are now a self-health / self-help nutritionist.

Congratulations!

You Are Now a Self-Health / Self-Help Sprouter!

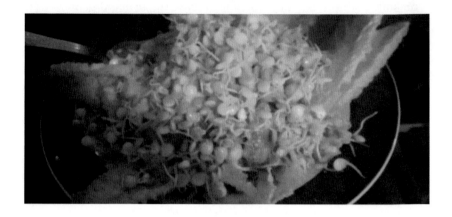

11: Closing Thoughts

This is not the last word on the subject of sprouting! It's designed to be the first words to help you get started and keep going!

You are in control of your health and nutrition. Take charge now by continuing to learn about every aspect of your nutritional world! So much of what we grew up with is toxic information about food and nutrition!

Feel free to try new seeds, grains, and beans to sprout. Always do some research to be sure it's a healthy choice.

Experiment with Your Sprouts

The internet has lots of great ideas for sprouts. Surf! Learn! Grow healthier!

Always shop around for the best deals! Prices vary greatly! I've seen alfalfa sprouts selling for $12 for 4 ounces in a health food store. I pay about $6 for a pound on eBay and from Now Foods for non-GM, organic seeds!

If you shop a variety of food stores, keep your eyes open in their pre-packaged bagged beans and their bulk bins... look for seeds and beans. Try them all! Pumpkin seeds are supposed to be wonderful sprouts... but I haven't tried them... yet... either!

Got Questions, Concerns?

...or Your Own Great Tips and Hints?

Tell Me! Feel free to contact me any time to discuss anything about the subject.

All I want is to live the healthiest, fullest life possible, maintaining optimum health and enjoying my days as best I can. My new lifestyle of sprouts, healthy food, and exercise has paid off in amazing rewards. I hope you enjoy similar results for yourself!

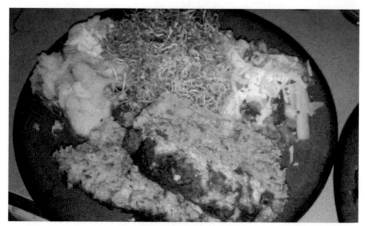

Veggie Loaf with Salad and Taters... Topped with Sprouts! Note: Veggie Loaf Made with Sprouts and Fiber from Juicing Veggies!

Appendix 1: More Info

About Sprouting, Sproute-rs, & Seeds

1. Internet Resources for <u>Sprouting: The Beginners Guide to Growing Sprouts!</u>

1. Facebook page devoted to this book, Facebook search for "Sprouting: The Beginners Guide to Growing Sprouts" or simply enter the URL, *https://www.facebook.com/pages/Sprouting-The-Beginners-Guide-to-Growing-Sprouts/644738185672813*

2. Our very own website / blog to help us all continue to grow with sprouting. www.BeginnersGuideToGrowingSprouting.com

2. Wikipedia

http://en.wikipedia.org/wiki/Sprouting

Great overview on sprouting and lots of good info to add to what you are getting here.

3. Food safety related to sprouts and sprouting.

http://www.foodsafety.gov/keep/types/fruits/sprouts.htm

<u>l</u>

Info from the government about food safety and sprouts and sprouting. Compared to the *guh-zillions* of people who die annually from the illnesses I managed to overcome, there is very little risk in sprouting. Check out this link. Then search for deaths from obesity, alone. Decide for yourself which route you want to take.

4. DetwilerNativeSeeds.

These are the guys who give everybody a great deal on alfalfa seeds. You can find them selling on eBay (www.eBay.com). Do a search for them, Detwilernativeseed. They have over 750 feedbacks and are over 99% positive. I got 3 pounds of organic alfalfa for $16 bucks (That included shipping FREE!).

I told them that I'd run out of alfalfa seeds and had waited too long to order. Without a hesitation, they expedited the shipment for me and got them to me in a couple of days! Very good folks there! And they really do want to help us all get better!

5. Products and Companies I Brag On!

If I'm bragging on a product or a company, it's because they've done right by me, plain and simple. When they go above and beyond, they get mentioned. If they slack

116

and cut corners, the bragging goes away. Send me your brags and I'll pass them along. We are here to help us all get better.

6. Amazon Seller: "Buy Wholesale Cheap"

I bought some great sprout mixes, by the pound, that were very nice and fairly affordable via Amazon. The seller is "Buy Wholesale Cheap." Look at their listings, they have sold tons of stuff and have great feedback ratings.

7. Search eBay and Amazon.

You can do a general search for "Sprout Seeds" and "Sprouter" to find great stuff to sprout and lots of different sprouters on both eBay and Amazon. Generally speaking, I've always found better deals on eBay and Amazon than from direct suppliers like the ones listed below. But they're all good at getting us what we want and need to heal and grow. I'm just a cheap guy... and friends don't let friends buy retail.

8. Mum's Sprouting Seeds

http://sprouting.com/

Another full range retail outfit for everything on the subject. Sprouters, sprouting seeds, supplies, and info. Free shipping on $75.00 orders. They are a bit rich for my wallet, but they've got it all, if you have the need and the cashola!

9. Sprout People

http://sproutpeople.org/

A full range supplier for everything related to sprouting. Retail. Pricing is a bit high for my tastes, too, but they do have "it all," and free shipping on orders over $60.

10. Many online vitamin and supplement sellers

Many online vitamin and supplement sellers carry a variety of sprouting seeds, too. Swanson's Vitamins has a few and since I get my supplements from them, I'll order a little something now and then since the shipping's free. Most of what they sell by way of sprouting seeds is Now Foods pre-packaged sprouting seeds.

11. Now Foods

Be sure to check with www.NowFoods.com to see

where you can find their sprouting products locally or nearby. I just went to their corporate website. They offer a one-pound zesty sprouting mix, containing clover, radish, and fenugreek, for just over six bucks a pound.

I plugged in my zip code and found a retailer about 2 miles from my home. I called the retailer. They only want $6.29 for a pound! Yep, Now Foods is my favorite corporate sprout dealer!!!! They don't get greedy and they make sure you can find it locally!

They sell smaller quantities of sprouting seeds in varieties that make it affordable to test new things.

Their sprouting jars are showing up at just about every natural food store I visit any more. I really like them and the price is just fine, about five bucks.

I can grow about a half gallon of sprouts in them. That gives me enough sprouts for 2 people for the four days it takes to get another batch grown.

12. Dried Beans

Dried beans are less likely to be sprayed with non-sprouting agents these days. I have gotten sproutable lentils from all the major grocers, including Wal-Mart and Target, in their dried bean section. Although Target is "Yuppifying" their grocery, so not sure if those beans will still be offered. Will update you as info comes in.

Same results go with chickpeas, AKA garbanzo beans.

13. Brick and Mortar Natural Grocers

National chains, like Whole Foods, Natural Grocers, and Central Market, as well as local and regional natural grocers carry a larger variety of bulk and pre-packaged organic seeds, grains, nuts, and legumes for sprouting. Organics are easy to find there!

Most of them I've been to in the past 2 years seem to carry the Now Foods sprouting jar at a good price. Many sell sprouting trays and other sprouting systems.

Prices have really come down for organics, too. It's great news for those of us who are trying to eat healthier.

14. Jim B the Presenter!

You can have Jim B present to your group or at your favorite natural food store. He brings sprouting samples with him and gives a great overview of the sprouting process! Jim's a fun and exciting presenter who clearly loves his calling! Contact him at Jim@KeepItSimplePublications.com

Appendix 2: About the Author

Jim Beerstecher (Jim B!)

The Sprouter! Jim B has been sprouting for thirty years, but only sporadically until the past 3 years. He's sprouted at home, on the road in his motorhome, at sea in his small sailboat, out camping, while visiting friends and relatives, and in hotel rooms.

Over the years, he'd let himself succumb to the American Industrial Food Complex and began to suffer the long-term effects of poor nutrition and diet. He was suffering from a number of chronic and potentially fatal illnesses, including: perforated diverticulitis, major depression, stage II hypertension, type II diabetes, morbid obesity, and arthritis.

He turned back to healthy whole foods, juicing, and sprouting! Today he's over 100 pounds lighter! Fit! Vigorous! He takes NO prescription medications! All of his chronic illnesses are gone!

Jim owes his amazing improvement to sprouting! And in this book he passes along what he's done, what he's learned, and everything you need to know to do the same!

All he asks in return is that you pass along what you learn and how it has helped you to the next person down the road who's suffering, too.

Appendix 3: Other Books by Jim B!

This is a catalog of the books by Jim B that are currently in print and available at Amazon and Jim B's websites: www.KeepItSimplePublications.com

Contact us at Inner Resources (dot biz) or Keep It Simple Publications (dot com) to arrange a personal appearance, book presentation, book signing, sprouting demonstration, or just to say, "Howdy!"

At Keep It Simple Publications dot com, we give you what you need to help YOU optimize your own inner resources!

SPROUTING: The Beginners Guide to Growing Sprouts!

Everything You Need to Know to Begin Growing & Enjoying Sprouts!

By Jim Beerstecher (Jim B)

Hey, didn't you just finish reading this book! : -

Enjoy great food, nutrition, and health for pennies! Here is everything you need to know to start growing delicious, affordable, tasty, healthy sprouts! All of that in a single jar! And working less than 5 minutes a week!

This is not the last word on the subject of sprouting! It's the first words to help you get started with sprouts and keep growing them!

In 2 years, Jim shed 100 pounds and has regained his health entirely. Here are the diagnoses he *no longer has*: perforated diverticulitis, type II diabetes, major depression, high blood pressure, sleep apnea, arthritis, acid reflux, and morbid obesity (or any obesity for that matter!). Jim was diagnosed with all those and had been obese for over 30 years!

And it all started with developing a simple, affordable, easy-to-use, ongoing, and health-restoring system for growing sprouts at home. For pennies, he began growing his own health and is today completely unrecognizable from the Jim of 2 years ago. No surgeries and no medications!

And it all started with a few sprouts grown on his kitchen counter... as it can for you. Once you see how simple, easy, and affordable it can be, you'll be on the road to better health, too!

Give this simple, affordable book a chance. Buy this book today! You have nothing to lose (Except weight, sickness, and misery!)and everything to gain!

Champagne Boating on a Beer Budget!

Buy and Equip Boats for Pennies on the Dollar! Save Thousands on Your Next Boat & the Boat Gear To Go with It!

By Jim Beerstecher

Why spend lots of money on a boat? With this fun and exciting text, you get the author's secrets to buying boats for pennies on the dollar!

Save time and money buying a boat and the gear to go with her! Get a boat now following these proven principles! Gives specific examples of boat deals the author has gotten and shares his hints and tips for getting similar deals on boats!

Updated to include all the internet sources and methodology you need to snap up a great deal on a boat! Jim's been buying sailboats for pennies on the dollar for over 30 years. Until now he's kept his secrets to himself. Now he's ready to retire and sail off forever, so he's sharing what he's learned!

Jim's helped lots of people find great boat deals and now he's going public with his knowledge. Get a great deal on a boat! Get a great deal on boat gear! Cut the dock lines and go cruising now! Why wait until you pay off a huge boat loan... Get a boat you can afford and go now!

For the cheap price of this book, you'll get a great return on your investment! Easily save a bundle on your next boat! *This is the book that boat brokers DON'T want you to read!*

Some boat deal's the author's found so far: A thirty foot

trimaran for $100; an Islander Bahamas 24 for $350; a Catalina 22, with trailer, for $600; a Venture 23 sailboat with trailer for $400; another Venture 23 with trailer with a new outboard motor for $200; a Bristol 24, for $600; an Islander 30 for $1900; and the ultimate coup (SO FAR!) a Hans Christian 34 for UNDER $5,000! *And then there are the free boats!*

Simply Brilliant Ideas & Projects for Sailboats & Power to Customize Your Boat and Prepare the Crew for Cruising!

Boatloads of Hints, Tips, and Great Ideas! To Save You Time, Money, and Problems!

By Jim Beerstecher

Must reading for people preparing to go cruising, whether power or sail! Helps you prepare your vessel, crew, pets, paperwork, galley, and money for the upcoming cruise! This book can save you buckets of dollars, too many hours of labor, and, tons of grief!

> **From the book...** *For forty-five years, you've lived a shore-based life. You understand things in your land-oriented world implicitly and rarely need to think about anything pertaining to your basic living circumstances. All of that's about to go flying out the window because YOU'RE getting ready to go cruising. You're entering into*

a new and foreign world. You need all of the help you can get to maximize the potential for success of your cruise.

A great source of knowledge about the cruising lifestyle comes from veteran cruisers, like Jim B! There are better sailors, out there! Jim B is an average cruiser with an average cruiser's lifetime experience and a lot of proven ideas to save you time, money, and energy!

The very few bucks spent here just might save your life someday! This book is a compendium of the boatloads of the slick things Jim B has learned along the way. That's what you need, basic hints, tips, and great ideas from a cruiser who's been there!

Any one hint, tip or idea is easily worth the price of this book and can enhance your cruising experience. ...and every copy you buy helps him stay out cruising just that much longer! Thanks!

Title: **Recovery: Passing Along Some Experience, Strength, and Hope!**

Subtitle: **A collection of 30 short stories related to recovery, life, living, and getting better.**

By Jim B

The author, who's been active in his own recovery since 1976, has pulled together some of his favorite stories about recovery.

He begins with his own story, "Jim B's Twelve Days of Christmas... a Miracle of Recovery." An alcoholic! A drug addict! A codependent! And a compulsive overeater! Jim's a good example of recovery being possible for the "*some of us are sicker than others*" crowd!

Good reading, fun accounts, anecdotes, slogans, sponsorship, meetings, steps, spirituality, treatment centers, old timers, relationships in recovery, employment, prosperity, and dozens of other components that make up a day in recovery are discussed. Something for everyone, new in recovery and old timers alike!

In this book, the author recounts some important and memorable lessons learned in his recovery. Each story will give the reader new insights into his/her own recovery. "If my readers gets one single new idea out of this book," quips Jim, "It's worth the price of admission and then some!"

Great gift idea! Great for people in any recovery program/s and for people who are contemplating joining a recovery program! It's a meeting in a digital format... got a few minutes? Glean some new perspectives for your own recovery!

Thank You from Inner Resources!

...And Thanks from Keep It Simple Publications!

We Want to Help You Improve

Your Own Inner Resources!

For More Information

Browse Our Website at

www.KeepItSimplePublications.com and/or
www.KeepItSimplePublications.com

email Jim@KeepItSimplePublications.com

To Order More Copies of this ebook at

Amazon.com, simply search "Jim Beerstecher" at
Amazon.com

Special thanks to CreateSpace and Kindle Direct Publishing for making this book possible in printed and ebook form!

Manufactured by Amazon.ca
Bolton, ON

27351060R00079